Clean Eating

40 Power Foods

Sudesh Abrol

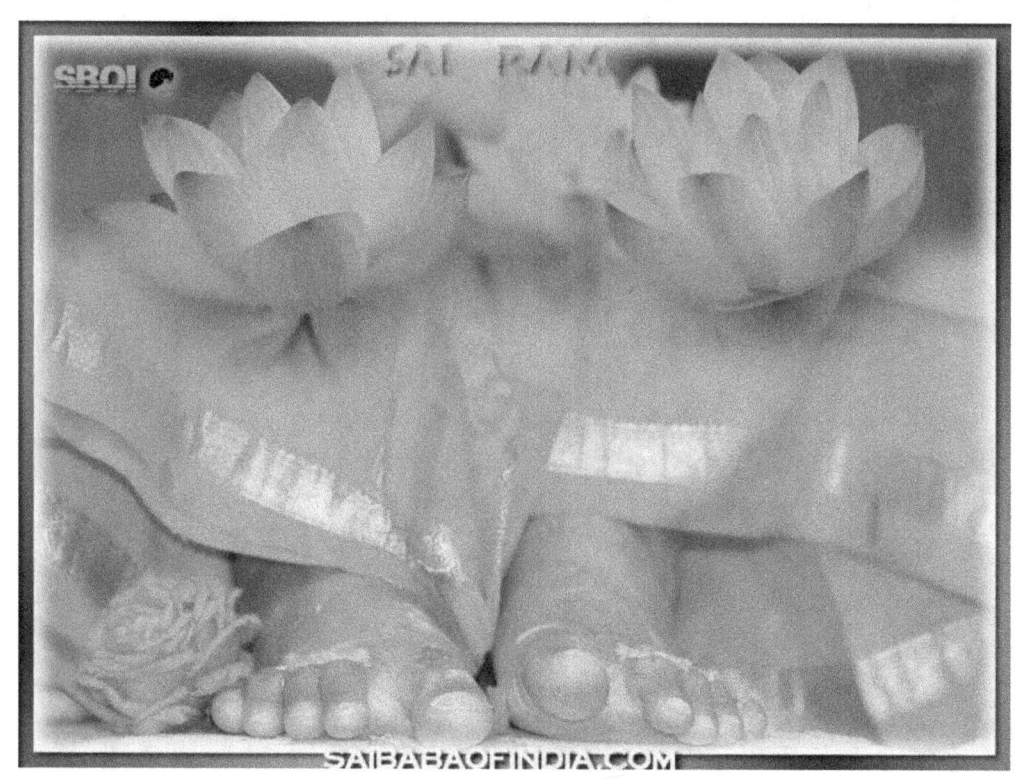

I am in thy Lotus feet always

Prepare a delicious meal for your loved ones that heals the body.

What others are saying about the Author:

It's never too late

I love the simplicity of this book! Sudesh gives common sense solutions to food and our mind that will help me be successful! This book should be 5 volumes, there is so much helpful information. I love the meditation! [By Annie Groth]

All in one book-how to live

I am a very health conscious lady who keeps reading all possible articles on health in different kind of books. Read this book again and again till I understood what this writer wants us to do with our body and I am surprised after reading this book how much I did not know. With my serious reading & my efforts to follow; my life has changed completely and I don't have to look for something else. "Peaceful Mind Skinny body" is like an ocean of knowledge. Thank you so much Sudesh Abrol for sharing so many things in such a simple way that everyone can understand and take advantage of your book. [by Uma Thukral / Kuwait]

A book to chew and digest

As Francis Bacon said, some books are to taste, others to be swallowed and some few to be chewed and digested; that is, some books are to be read only in parts; others to be read, but not curiously; and some few to be read wholly, and with diligence and attention. This book by Sudesh Abrol definitely falls in the latter category. It is a well written and well thought out book. Can't wait for the next addition! [By Dr. Harpreet Jaswal]

A very beneficial book to read

If you want real health advice rather than the cliché advice that you always hear, I highly suggest this book. I definitely have a different perspective of what "peace" is now for my mind and body, and can live a stress-free life. A plus is that I also look and feel healthier.

Peaceful Mind, Skinny Body

All I have to say is Thank You for sharing your knowledge!! This book has taught me how easy it is to live a healthy lifestyle. Once I understood this, the weight just melted away. This book is the best investment I've made in my future and the future of my family! [By Seema Lopez]

Prepare a great meal that satiates your palate, nurtures your mind and nourishes your soul.

Contents

Preface

Food is the fuel that powers our lives, a source of nutrients and gives energy to the body to carry out our daily internal and external functions. We all are supposed to believe that's what food should be.

Unfortunately in today's modern age, many of us consume far too many packaged and processed foods that fail to give us the life-sustaining nutrients our body needs. Those individuals, who eat healthy food still have problems processing the nutrients required to stay healthy, energized, active and vibrant.

Plant based foods and nuts provide the most benefits in their natural form. Vegetables which you cannot eat raw, you may steam or cook a little crunchy to protect the nutrients. If you overcook vegetables to make the food tastier, then you are depriving your body of the nutrients, minerals and enzymes.

If you use a lot of butter/oil in your cooking to make it delicious, then it is unlikely you will lose weight and stay healthy, rather it is likely you will gain weight. You can bake, sauté, cook or steam the vegetables with salt, turmeric, and black pepper; then sprinkle olive oil or coconut oil over it and enjoy your meal. Be a little creative when you prepare your delicious recipes.

The goal of life is to be healthy, active and vibrant. For a fit and healthy body, we can consume alkaline foods which prevent mental and physical disorders. Non-alkaline foods generate acidity, which is notorious for creating gas, and can be the start of dangerous conditions in the body. Here are a few alkaline foods: All dairy products, butter, most nuts such as almonds, hazelnuts, walnuts, chestnuts and Brazil nuts.

Fruits, juicy fruits, fruit juices and especially fresh home-made juice; apples, apricots, bananas, pineapples, water-rich foods such as watermelons and all kinds of berries, figs and papayas, all come from this category. Avocados, tomatoes, and lemons are also salty foods and are highly recommended to neutralize acidity. Well-ripped berries are an excellent food, but if they are raw they produce fermentation, and all acidic foods generate bitterness, which eventually leads to diseases. Soybean is the most alkaline food, and it helps as a treatment for acidity.

Soy products are available in the market as flour, nuggets, granules and ready-made soybeans products. These are high in protein. Most vegetables are alkaline, especially all the greens, like broccoli, kale, spinach, zucchini, and cabbage, and we can use all kinds of vegetables in our everyday life to keep us healthy. In my recipe books, 'Scrumptious Meals from India,' in the different volumes, you can find several interesting and delicious recipes, which you may easily cook yourself at home. There are many kinds of luscious soup recipes, which assist in cleansing the skin, intestines, stimulate the digestive system, and help lose weight. All these vegetables are full of nutrients, vitamins, enzymes, fiber and minerals. You can eat soup as much as you desire because these soups will satiate your pallet, fill you up, and help you shed some pounds. These are fat cutter soups.

It is important you read the entire book and find the foods which work best for your body. You can pick those items and make a chart of those you will be consuming on a regular basis. You may also plan an adequate portion for your daily meals. Remember, all the greens you will eat are free foods. That means even if you eat a little extra, you will gain no weight. So, feel free and enjoy all the greens available in the market. Be little creative, cook your food with love and dedication and enjoy delicious meals. This food has to be delicious because you are not feeding your body alone; you are also nourishing your soul.

Please do not starve and miss a single meal. It is essential to keep your metabolism active. If you miss a meal, thinking you will lose some weight faster, then this is a wrong perception. It slows down metabolism; one suffers from poor elimination; the system starts accumulating fat, weight, and toxins, which later develops in generating bacteria and turning it into a disease. Never miss your breakfast, because a healthy breakfast prepares you to face the challenges of the day. While feeding your body – you are serving your SOUL residing within.

Introduction

When a car accident in 1984 left her in acute pain with spinal damage, Sudesh started medical treatment which involved years of medication consumption, physical therapy, and epidural injections. The severe pain still persisted! She was told by several doctors that she would have to live with the pain.

Her nephew, who was a Yoga Expert and a Naturopath, was visiting from India. He introduced her to several Yoga postures that decreased the pain by at least 30%. He also gave her herbs from the kitchen. Sudesh went to India in 1988 and learned more about Yoga, Pranayam, Meditation, and Nature Cure from the renowned teachers and guru in the hills of Himalayas. Her writings in her books reflect the knowledge that she has attained. As a senior citizen, she can proudly profess that her pain has diminished completely! She strongly believes, "We are what we eat." She lives disease-free. She is not dependent on any medications and she is thankful to the Lord for the life she is blessed with.

Sudesh is constantly asked about her diet regiment and this book is a gift for those "Who want to know"! There is no secret in what she consumes. The discipline lies within the daily choices she makes!

Aging Gracefully

Aging gracefully is a blessing. In the present time, life is so busy and hectic that each and every one feels mental stress and body tension. Stress is the primary cause of feeling and making us old before time, and old age is a curse. My friend always gets upset when she looks in the mirror and questions, "Who is this person in the mirror, do I know her?" Why do we get old faster? Is it a natural process of life or we are doing something wrong? Honestly speaking no one wants to be old, and no one wishes to look past.

In fact, we are demanding too much from life. We need to put a ceiling on our desires. Therefore, it is essential to calm the mind and discipline the body with the best tools like Yoga, Pranayam and Meditation. Millions of people are suffering from the severe disorder of stress; staying home and have no jobs or do not want to work. Losing interest in life also makes us feel and look old and worthless.

Let us adopt a few simple habits; change the lifestyle, and live a young, active and vibrant life without spending any money. Smile at everyone you see or meet and let the anger go. A smile is contagious. If you see someone without smiling, give one of yours. Every day set priorities to avoid stress and disappointments. Have a quest for learning new things instead of complaining. Become a good listener instead of talking too much and wasting valuable energy. Judge less and accept more. Trust in your "SELF." Fear not and love everyone. We adapt good habits of chewing food properly, an adequate portion of food, and consuming more alkaline foods that help to avoid having disorders. Also, we can eat maximum food in natural form. Also to stay active and vibrant, it is advisable to incorporate 15 minutes cardio exercise each day; thus having no weight problem.

Invest a little sincere effort in yoga, pranayam and meditation daily for your wellness and staying healthy; you will be able to eliminate and solve many of your problems yourself. This regular practice helps you experience feeling young, being healthy mentally, physically and spiritually. Life is beautiful, and life is happiness. Please do not look out for peace and happiness. Joy and peace are already inside you. You have to do little effort yourself; explore inside you, and awaken your potential. You can receive the reward of the secrets of the Gurus and Masaya to cultivate your body and nourish your soul. And remember, only meditation will help you to reach your goal.

And now I am going to tell you the secret of living healthy, looking young and being always cheerful and active. Eating a healthy small portion of food, working hard mentally and physically, sleeping short hours and smiling all the time is the super-secret formula to look and stay young. You think I am kidding? No, this is written in our ancient spiritual scriptures and also our Gurus teach us so. That is the reason I thank The Supreme Power for giving me this lifestyle. I thank those Gurus and Acharyas, whom I met in the Kumaon hills and mountains of the Himalayas in India for giving me all this knowledge, not to abuse this body, stay young, healthy, happy and vibrant.

Obesity

Statistics confirm that the US has the most obese people of all nations. The biggest cause for obesity is fast food. Food manufacturers do not care about the ingredients they put in their food. Their goals are to cook tasty food and to maximize revenue. Their focus is on your money, nothing else. When you buy fast food, do you ever check label for fat, calories, and sodium contents? If you learn the truth, you will be amazed at the statistics.

The second biggest reason for obesity is the eating habits of the parents. Obese parents continue to raise their kids by the same patterns of eating they have adopted for themselves. They enjoy large portions of high-calorie foods, deserts, and pre-packaged foods. These ready-made foods contain very little fiber and essential nutrients. The foods being stored in their stomachs may also contribute to impotency in men and women. In addition, in later life, these foods cause the liver to weaken and, as a result, people suffer from diabetes, constipation, acidity, intestinal problems, and high blood pressure. They omit nutrients, fiber, and mother's love, which she adds while cooking the food. I strongly believe that eating light foods five times a day with a well-balanced low-fat diet-plan and proper portions, as well as participating in regular vigorous exercise with weights six days a week for 15 minutes daily, you will lose weight and enjoy a healthy and vibrant body. Home cooked meals and exercise are important for the body.

I have seen mothers who over feed their children. When the children grow up with extra weight, the same mothers worry and lie, saying their children do not eat anything and still are gaining weight. I would like to advise all mothers: "You are the first teacher, discipline your babies with proper portions of food, do not baby sit them 24/7; teach them simple habits, and let them grow as normal kids." Forcing food on your children due to your overwhelming love may damage your child's future. Children know nothing, and tend to eat more than the capacity of their hunger. Therefore, it is your duty to regulate your child's life, and not to let them munch on food the entire day.

People with Depression are more likely to be overweight. They stay home, watch TV, eat frequently, and have no interest in life or anything. They do not cook, and live a lazy life. They over-eat due to their depression. They love ready-made food and eat more than they require.

How a person wants to live depends upon the individual. Everything is within you, divinely installed. You have to put in the effort to help yourself and fix yourself. With the help of yoga, breathing exercises, and meditation, you can awaken your inner potential and find the abundance. · To lose weight, drink 40 oz. of water early in the morning and eat no food for one hour. If constipated, drink warm water with a half teaspoon of salt. Drinking warm water helps to set your metabolism, clean your intestinal track, and eliminate constipation. We call the procedure Usha Paan (Aqua Therapy), and it is a Yoga based natural cure.

When you decide to live healthy, do not settle for one item or a few things; it makes life dull and boring. Get into a regular habit of consuming a variety of these different kinds of foods on a daily basis to heal your body. Eat to your satisfaction, lose weight, and lead a healthy life. Be creative and cook with the spices of your choice, adding onions, ginger, garlic, tomatoes and green peppers. Make a delicious dish that satisfies your pallet. The aim of our life has to be 'living healthy,' because it is your birthright. For me, my health is a treasure, I want you to enjoy a healthy body and live happy and in peace Consult your doctor before you start eating any new vegetable on a daily basis because some vegetables are high in some compounds and vitamins such as Vitamin K that can interrupt your medications, especially if you have a heart condition and are taking medicine like Warfarin.

Aloe Vera

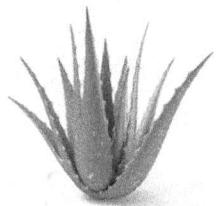

Aloe Vera is an excellent short-stemmed plant that possesses water in its leaves, and the entire world is familiar with it. Because of its therapeutic properties, people will love to keep this plant in their homes when they know that this is like having a doctor in the house! Some people know its benefits and grow aloe vera plants in the kitchen. Aloe vera keeps the environment clean, and secretes a lot of oxygen which we the humans need. Carbon dioxide, which we exhale, gets absorbed by the plant immediately. Many people, like me, keep a pot of aloe vera on the kitchen counter near the window. The gel squeezed from aloe vera leaf, contributes to give relief for minor wounds and burns. Its thick juice from the leaf supports as the skin softening agent. Modern manufacturers and reputed companies are using it in their creams, shampoos, lotions and masks and proudly populate on their products "made with pure aloe vera." There is an estimated annual market of $14 billion globally.

Flatulence: Aloe vera gel possesses most of the bioactive compounds in the stems. It also contains vitamins, antioxidants, enzymes, amino acids, and minerals. Remove the pointy thorns of the skin of 2" of aloe vera stem, chop and boil it in half a cup of water. If you consume it daily, this contributes to helping chronic flatulence.

Bad Breath and Teeth: If someone can chew on a 1" clean piece of aloe vera and swallow it each day, it will assist to kill bad breath and maintain the health of your teeth. But please remember that aloe vera plant is bitter, whereas some are not. How do I know this? Because I have both varieties!

Helps Acne Skin: If you are suffering from acne problems, then massage a drop of aloe vera jelly gently on the affected area. It aids to dry acne faster.

Dry Skin: Mix one teaspoon of aloe vera jelly and half a teaspoon of pure almond oil. Apply on your face, neck or hands, and you will experience a great feeling of an excellent moisturizer to tone and condition your skin. Continuous use of this great homemade moisturizer will help your face, neck, and hands look soft and smooth, healthy and young.

Helps Diabetes: Aloe Vera plant includes medicinal therapy properties and in Ayurvedic herbal medicines, aloe vera plays a significant role. In Nature Cure, aloe vera juice is given to diabetic patients every day, and we also use the gel for many different physical problems.

Skin Eruptions: People used aloe vera frequently for external application to heal open wounds, irritation, and bruises in ancient times. In Nature Cure treatment, its leaf extract is given to people as a tonic for those who suffer from jaundice. It can regenerate the damaged tissues. This gel may also be consumed to aid flush out toxins of the body.

Inflammation: The medicinal therapy compounds appear in aloe vera, contribute to decreasing inflammation in the body. Due to certain allergies, some individuals get their body parts swelled up, but with the regular consumption of aloe vera gel twice a day, supports to reduce the swelling.

Some people can easily handle aloe vera and some cannot. I have talked to my friends, relatives, my yoga students and several other people, who told me their experiences and methods of consuming it. Some can take one inch piece of fresh aloe vera, peel off the prickly-edged thorns and skin and cut the transparent gel into tiny pieces. They wrap it in one tablespoon of yogurt or one teaspoon of honey and swallow in one gulp with a cup of water.

Another way is, to clean one inch piece of fresh aloe vera, and take it with water. I clean it, prick the thick gel with the fork and take with water. It has become a habit now. Do you know what I do with the two pieces of aloe vera peels? I apply the liquid gel of the peels on my face and neck and let it dry. It assists my skin to look smooth, clean, tight and toned. I always welcome free treatments.

I would love to share the amazing experience I had with aloe vera. Two years ago, I made homemade tablets with aloe vera and amla powder. In the US, people know amla as amlika. It is available in oriental, Indian and herbal stores. I took three aloe vera leaves and let them drained the yellow juice overnight (as my yoga instructor had advised me). Next morning, I washed them, peeled them and cut them into pieces. I made the gel in the blender and put it in the sun to dry. I mixed the amla powder and one spoon of starch as a binder and made pea size tablets. I put the pills in a large flat tray with dry flour so not to stick to each other and put them to dry in the sun. My husband and I were taking these tablets every day as it helped cleanse the blood. One tablet each a.m. and p.m. My granddaughter, who was eighteen had acute acne problems on her face and was getting treatment from a professional dermatologist. I told her to take these tablets but, because they looked weird, she refused to take and also she had never swallowed any medicine before. One day while giving her a facial, I convinced her that if she took those tablets every day, that would help her. She agreed and started taking them. When we met after two weeks at a family get together, I was amazed to see her face as it had started clearing up, and she looked gorgeous. Since then my other grandkids also started consuming these homemade tablets. As I said before, aloe vera helps to push out toxins out of the body. I make jelly of two stems of aloe vera and refrigerate it in a bottle. I use it very often on cuts, burns, and face. I also swallow one tablespoon of it with water in the morning (empty stomach)and massage my face with it for 30 seconds.

How to make the gel? When you separate the stems from the plant, leave them in the sink overnight, and let the yellow juice drain out. This yellow color substance is not edible. The next day, wash the stems with a brush because it has sharp prickly-edged thorns and slice them off carefully. It possesses a thick transparent gel inside. The gel looks awesome, but it is bitter. Some plants are not too bitter.

Amla

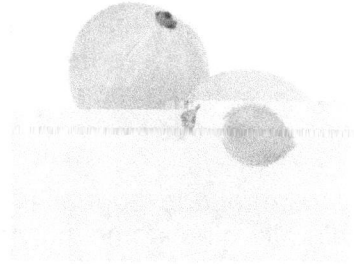

Amla is so beneficial that its fruit, bark, and leaves are used to make powders, face packs and juices to treat the body. Here are the benefits of amla which will amaze you to discover why we call it a "Miracle Fruit."

Do we all want our locks to be lustrous & long? Yes, we all do! Lustrous, thick, shiny, long and healthy hair like those shampoo models in the magazines and on TV, are a dream for all of us. Indian Gooseberry or Amla is a very famous herb or fruit in India. Amla, also known as Amlika here in the USA, is a miracle fruit and makes an excellent recipe get those long thick, lustrous hair back. Amla is an excellent pickled companion that makes the main course delicious; it also makes a great recipe to get those long locks back. We lose a lot of hair due to many reasons that we may not even realize. The number one reason is mental and physical stress, and also, hair stress is a common factor when we expose our hair to certain factors such as using more shampoo, chemicals in hair dyes and special heat treatments. I advise only one of the most recommended ways to rejuvenate your hair is by using amla regularly.

For Lustrous Hair: Soak a quarter cup of dry amla in half a cup of water overnight. Wash your hair with the amla water massaging the scalp thoroughly twice a week. This amla juice penetrates the skin, nourishes and strengthens the follicles. It increases the natural beauty of your hair and makes dandruff disappear. In India, women dye their hair with the mixture of henna, coffee, and dry amla powder. They make a paste, apply to the hair and leave it in for hours. Their hair looks shining, thick and lustrous.

Cures Stress: Washing hair with amla helps remove stress; it has a cooling effect on eyes and brain, and you enjoy a peaceful sleep at night. Being so sour, it can clean the hair properly, and no shampoo is needed.

Fight Free Radicals And Maintain Youthfulness: Amla is the powerhouse of anti-oxidants and helps to fight off free radicals in the human body. Regular consumption of amla powder or juice reduces the risk of many horrible diseases. It works as pro-biotic. One can maintain youthfulness with daily use of amla. When I was studying Nature Cue in India, at Rishikesh Ashram in the hills of Himalaya, my Acharyas always said, "Eat amla every day and plush old age away." I believe it is true.

Help Push Out Toxins: Prepackaged and processed food, fried, and sugary food, intoxicating beverages, modern medicines, etc. regularly increases the buildup of a large amount of toxins in our body. Amla helps in maintaining the proper function of kidneys, liver and bladder, and the removal of the toxins. One teaspoon of amla powder on an empty stomach every morning will do the work.

Rich Source of Vitamin C: Amla is an excellent source of vitamin C. Consume one teaspoon of amla powder every day, and you do not need vitamin C supplements that are not readily absorbed by the body.

Cures Cold and Sore Throat: Consumption of one teaspoon of amla powder mix with one teaspoon of honey first thing in the morning helps heal a cold and a sore throat. Repeat four times a day for great results.

Removes Constipation: Daily consumption of one teaspoon of amla powder removes constipation problem. Amla is rich in fibers, works as a gentle laxative and makes bowel movement smooth.

Heels Mouth Cankers: If you suffer from mouth cankers frequently then, swallow one teaspoon of amla powder at bedtime for four days. Also, dilute a quarter cup of the amla juice in half a cup of water and gargle with this mixture daily for positive results.

Heals Arthritis stiffness and Pain: Is Amla beneficial in reducing arthritis stiffness and pain? It has anti-inflammatory properties that help in reducing stiffness, swelling and joint pain. Consume raw amla or its juice daily in the morning diluted in water twice a day. If fresh amla or juice is not available, then you can use one teaspoon of amla powder twice a day for one month and once daily for at least two months.

Improves Eyesight: Amla is very useful to enhance eyes health and eyesight. It also reduces redness, itching, stickiness and watering. Mix 2 teaspoons of amla juice in half a cup of water and drink it every morning. Dilute one teaspoon of amla juice in a quarter cup of water and with the help of an eye cup cleanse your eyes every morning leaving Amla water in the eyes for 5 to 6 seconds.

Helps Cure Sleeping Disorder: If you don't sleep well, then try this "magic fruit" to relieve stress and enjoy a good night sleep. Consume a teaspoon of amla powder each morning before consuming anything and do not eat anything for 30 minutes.

Regulates Acidity Level In Digestive System: Regular consumption of amla helps balance the acidity level in the stomach. It also stimulates the power of digesting food thus improving the digestive system.

Helps Stimulate Metabolism and Lose Weight: If you are suffering from a sluggish digestive system, then Amla will help to stimulate your metabolism and you may lose some weight.

Strengthens Respiratory And Central Nervous System: Amla helps strengthen the lungs, the respiratory system and the nervous system of your body.

Boosts Immunity: Now scientists are predicting that vitamin C will be the future medicine for many physical disorders. Daily consumption of an amla or a teaspoon of its powder helps boost immunity due to its high contents of vitamin C.

Purifies Blood And Improves Hemoglobin: Amla purifies blood and increases the hemoglobin level in the blood. I remember my mom made me drink diluted amla juice when I was a teenager because I had acne problems. It is helpful for skin problems also.

Maintains Cholesterol: Looking for natural alternatives for high cholesterol? High cholesterol (LDL) may trigger the probability of a heart attack or a stroke. Amla helps cleanse the clogging in the arteries of the heart. Take a teaspoonful of amla powder daily with a glass of water twice a day before meals. It will help to lower your numbers when you visit your doctor after consuming, at least, three months. You will also be happy to see your good cholesterol (HDL) increased significantly.

Apples

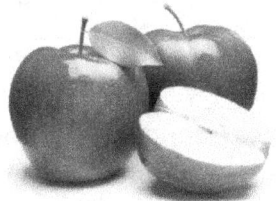

Why are apples so in demand?

Apples are full of fiber. They contain a special kind of fiber called pectin, and an apple of medium size has approximately 4 grams of fiber. Pectin fiber works on our body repairing our health in many areas. In the year 2004, USDA scientists researched over 100 foods to find their antioxidant concentration per serving size. They found red delicious and granny smith apples were ranked 12th and 13th respectively. Antioxidants are the compounds that fight diseases in the body and scientists believe these compounds help repair and prevent the damage done by the oxidation during normal cell activity.

Healthier and Whiter Teeth: When you bite and chew an apple, it stimulates the production of saliva in your mouth and reduces tooth decay by lowering the level of bacteria. If your teeth are dissolving, hurting or gums swell up, start eating a large sized apple before two main meals regularly.

Helps Avoid Alzheimer's Disease: Doctors and we people in Nature Cure believe that drinking apple juice can help fight Alzheimer away and the effects of aging on the brain. But remember, I am talking about 'fresh apple juice' as a regular diet for those who have Alzheimer in the family or if you know someone who is showing signs of it. You can also encourage your children if they are not bringing good grades and forgetting things quickly, to eat one large unpeeled apple 10 minutes before eating two meals. They have to chew it slowly and correctly and watch the positive results.

Helps Lower Cholesterol: The soluble fiber found in apples helps lower the cholesterol level. It also stimulates the digestive system and the intestines which make the smooth bowel movement. You enjoy a feeling of 'a healthier you'.

Help Curb All Kinds of Cancers: Scientists from the American Association for Cancer Research and Naturopaths agree the consumption of apples on a daily basis can contribute to reducing your risk of developing different kinds of cancers. Apple peels contain several compounds that have the potential to disable the cancer cells in the liver, breast and colon. The frequent intake of apples with the skin also helps to reduce the risk of colorectal cancer, but one has to chew it slowly and thoroughly for the best results.

Healthier heart: Plaque builds inside the arteries which reduces blood flow to the heart. This leads to coronary artery disease and there may be the chances of getting a heart attack or a stroke. Eating two apples a day religiously with the peel helps to prevent plaque buildup around the arteries because the skin contains high soluble fiber. This soluble fiber also contributes to preventing the cholesterol that gets into the human system and solidifies on the artery walls. The delicious apple jam (with less sugar) helps give energy if the patient feels week or is in heart sinking condition.

Decrease Risk of Diabetes: People who eat one apple very day have fewer chances of getting diabetes. The soluble fiber is so useful for the digestive system that it does not let sugar get too high. Try to consume green apples as they have lots of soluble fibers and will help the blood sugar to stay at a healthy level.

Prevent Kidney Stones: Kidney stones are the product of the kidney. These stones are taken out with the operation but in spite of this, these stones are formed again. Drinking apple juice has been found to eliminate the formation of stones, and if they are already in your system this juice helps it break down, and it comes out through the urine tract. Apple juice contributes to clean the kidney and removes the kidney stone pain. Even if you eat apples for a few days, it helps to eliminate kidney stones. If you still need more food, try to consume more apples and vegetables.

Eliminate Constipation and Diarrhea: If you eat apples as breakfast, it eliminates constipation. If you are constipated then eat apples with the peel, it also helps to cure diarrhea. If you consume food rich in fiber that helps stomach problems and try to avoid fatty foods and dairy products.

Avoid Hemorrhoids: The consumption of high fibrous food like apples can help reduce hemorrhoids pain.

Control your weight: Fruits like apples and vegetables with high fiber can help you to monitor your weight that will help you from various diseases like heart disease, stroke, and high blood pressure. You will also improve your overall health.

Detoxify your liver: The consumption of apples empowers your liver to detoxify easily.

Ashwagandha

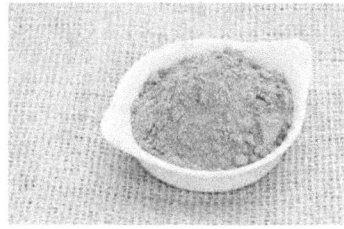

Ashwagandha is a very popular herb in the whole world and also known as 'Indian Ginseng.' It is available all over India, but especially in the Himalaya region in the dry lands and on the height of over 5000 ft. It comes in many varieties, and only the experts choose these herbs for their active medicinal purposes. The experts recognize ashwagandha by its peculiar strong smell only when they crush it. Ashwagandha possesses highly beneficial properties. We can consume it with other herbs also. We use its powder and swallow half a spoon of ashwagandha powder with water in the morning of evening. It is herbalists' favorite herb, and they are utilizing it with many herbal and Ayurvedic medicines for over 3000 years. It is the world's great herb root; has a broad range of activity that promotes physical and mental health, boosts longevity, and rejuvenates the body.

Helps Joint Pains: Because of its inflammatory benefits, it aids to reduce inflammation in the body and joints, soothes joint and arthritis pain and improves overall physical health. I had a car accident in 1984 and suffered from spine damage for 28 years. No doctor here in the US could fix me. I was in India in 2011 and a great Swamiji, who lives in the Himalaya mountains, told me to consume Giloye, Amla, and ashwagandha powders early in the morning. I have eaten these three herbs together for a couple of years and now live with no disease in my body.

Helps Maintain Youth: Ashwagandha is full of antioxidants, inflammatory compounds and saints and seers understand its value very well. They consume it fresh or its powders and extracts, as they live in mountains, and they know where it grows; they look ageless. It provides strength, energy and improves vitality. It also promotes longevity. I have consumed it for a couple of years as a pro-biotic to stay healthy.

Helps Anxiety: Ashwagandha has high contents of antioxidant compounds and is very famous for contributing calmness and improving energy.

Helps Fertility: In India, herbalists give ashwagandha powder or extract to many men and women as a treatment to promote healthy fertility. Ashwagandha is famous for its stimulating effects on fertility.

Helps Energy: Numerous fresh energy products, like energy chews, gel packets, energy powders, and sports drinks that promote health and physical fitness, are available in the market, but they only provide extra calories and do nothing actually to support physical ability. In 2012, India's Guru Nanak Dev University's Sports Medicine and Physiotherapy conducted an eight weeks study in which expert long drive cycle users supplemented with ashwagandha and at the end of the study they found significant enhancements in both cardiovascular and respiratory endurance.

Helps Alzheimer's: Because of the high medicinal properties of Ashwagandha, it is very helpful to the patients suffering from Alzheimer. It not only boosts their energy but also improves a physical weakness. It also aids to sharpen memory. When I was learning Yoga and Nature Cure in India at one of the Ashrams, where children with little less ability were also there for the treatment with their parents, they were learning breathing exercises, how to focus and were regularly getting a dose of ashwagandha with honey, lemon, and some other herbs. It has also been proven, if school-going children, who are slow in studies, can improve their grades if they consume Ashwagandha powder on a regular basis. In Ayurvedic medicine, the primary use of ashwagandha root extract is, to enhance memory and to improve brain function.

Helps with Chemotherapy: Research out of Malaysia found when patients consumed ashwagandha root extract regularly while receiving chemotherapy; it had the potential to relieve the related fatigue, increase energy, and improve their quality of life.

Helps Relieve Stress: Stress affects both mind and body and can be a strain that leads to depression. Most people will also agree tension and stress reduce the quality of life. Herbalists believe that_ashwagandha has properties to fight the pressure. Greek and Ayurvedic medicines have documented it for its stress reducing properties.

Helps Common Colds and Flu: Ashwagandha is a marvelous herb that can heal diabetes, cough, flu and many more physical conditions. Its antioxidants and high potency of inflammatory contents are very beneficial for the common cold, allergies, and the flu. Even heart patients get ashwagandha for treatment, but you do not take it until you check with your physician.

NOTE: - Before starting to adopt a new herb or medicine, you must consult your doctor for the advice. Ashwagandha may cause drowsiness or if you are taking any medications that could interact with their effects. Sometimes you cannot take herbs with the modern medicines, so it is advisable to check with your doctor.

Avocado

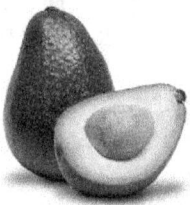

The avocado is a unique kind of fruit, and I had never seen it in India, but now it is available everywhere. Most fruits consist of carbohydrates, whereas avocado has healthy low carbs and includes healthy fats. Several studies show it has excellent benefits for health. Here are some healthy benefits of avocado, which are supported by Naturopaths and the scientists. It is very popular for its fresh flavor and rich texture. Avocado is the main ingredient in the most popular dish guacamole. Because of its health properties and high nutrients, it has become a favorite of everyone and now is known as super food. There are different kinds of avocados out there, but the most famous ones are called Hass avocados. Avocados are free of sodium and cholesterol. It contains 15 grams of healthy fats, about 150 calories, 2 grams of protein and my friends call it a low-carb friendly plant food and I call it a delicious food. It consists of healthy fats, lot of fiber and many nutrients. Avocado Is an incredibly nutritious Fruit.

Calms Arthritis and Osteoarthritis Pain: Arthritis and Osteoarthritis are enormous common problems in this world. I have witnessed several young as well as matured persons suffering from arthritis. Arthritis is also in variety with many names, and people believe that they have this problem for the rest of their lives, but it is not true. If you have belief on nature cure, then live with nature, consume natural foods that help to heal your body and bones and get some relief. I believe Mother Nature has the abundance for us. Avocados are helpful for osteoarthritis and arthritis patients. Half an avocado if consumed every day, lubricates the joints and helps decrease pain.

Stables Blood pressure: Avocado contains high potassium, and Potassium is a crucial mineral for the body. Many people do not get enough potassium in their food. This mineral helps support healthy blood pressure level, strengthens the body, the body cells, and serves various important functions.

Avocado is a high-fat food, but remember, this fat is natural and healthy, and the human body absorbs it faster. Avocado comes with a monounsaturated fatty acid; also this major component is found in olive oil and we all know and believe in its beneficial effects. It is full of fiber, which is also a major compound for the body.

Lose Weight: The fiber in avocado stimulates the digestive system and helps to maintain weight. Being good carbs, it gives you a feeling of fullness, and you do not feel hungry soon after. I have seen people consuming one avocado at breakfast daily. Containing healthy low carbs and high fiber, it helps us to promote lose weight.

Heart Health: Avocado is a heart healthy food, and it helps strengthen heart muscle. You can eat one-half avocado every day (with your physician's consent) as a pro-biotic to stay healthy. Researchers show avocados can improve heart disease and enhance the health of a heart patient.

Lower Cholesterol: Avocado helps lower cholesterol level (LDL) and triglyceride numbers if regularly consumed. It also helps in inflammatory conditions and one may find an increase in HDL. I have friends who are on a low-fat vegetarian diet. They eat half an avocado every day and are maintaining their cholesterol, weight, and energy.

Healthy for Cancer Patients: Avocados do not contain any fat, but the majority of the fat in it is oleic acid. This oleic acid helps to reduce inflammation in the body. It also contributes to strengthening the organs and body tissues, but it helps the cancer cells, I have not heard. A few of my students told me they felt safe when they ate one avocado daily during their chemotherapy. Avocado oil is also very beneficial and is considered safe for cooking. I love to eat half an avocado every day and enjoy guacamole very often.

Helps Eyes: Avocados hold powerful antioxidants that can help protect our eyes and strengthen eye muscles. Researchers tell us that avocados can also reduce the risk of cataracts and macular degeneration, which is a very common problem in the old generations. The high level of antioxidants in it helps the absorption of nutrients from other foods.

Helps Diabetes: Avocado being healthy low-carbs plant food, helps diabetic patients to maintain their sugar level. Getting into a new habit of consuming half an avocado every day will improve your health, weight, and sugar level and you will notice a feeling of being healthy.

Mixing avocado with your salsa, salads, adding to a sandwich or making guacamole will not only increase antioxidant absorption when you consume every day, but you will also notice you own an active and healthy body. BUT IF YOU HAVE A THYROID CONDITION, TRY TO STAY AWAY FROM IT.

Barley

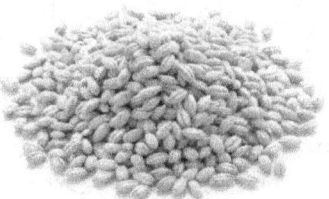

Whole grain foods have quickly been gaining popularity over the past few years. Barley grain is on the top. There are many other grains like Millet, Ragi, Jowar, Corn, and wheat, but barley is the number one grain for its various health benefits. Now doctors also recommend consuming cereals. Whole grains are essential sources of dietary fiber, vitamins, and minerals that are not available in refined and enriched grains. It is a versatile cereal grain with a rich nutty flavor, and one has to chew it properly. Though it looks like wheat berries, yet it is slightly lighter in color. Sprouted barley is profoundly good, and the manufacturers use grain to make beer and other alcoholic beverages.

It is available in two forms: one is hulled, slightly processed to remove only the inedible outer shell, leaving the germ and bran intact. The second is barley pearls, and you will not find the layer of bran and the hull. Pearl barley is very popular in the US, but hulled barley is higher in fiber and nutrition because the bran layer is left intact.

Half a cup of hulled barley contains 325 calories, 11 grams of protein, 2 grams of fat and 0 cholesterol. It has 65 grams of carbohydrates and 16 grams of dietary fiber. It has been found to lower insulin resistance and blood cholesterol levels thus helping us to reduce the risk of obesity and provide an immunity boost.

It is the belief that consuming plant-based foods of all variety can contribute to reducing the risk of many health problems. Many studies have suggested that increasing consumption of plant foods such as barley decreases the likelihood of heart disease, obesity, diabetes, and promotes a healthy complexion and thick hair, increased energy, and overall lower weight.

Blood Pressure: Consuming barley every day helps to lower the blood pressure. I grind barley and other grains in my coffee grinder and make pancakes, salty pancakes with onions and green chilies. I soak steel-cut oats with the whole pearl barley at night and in the morning I cook for 15 minutes on medium heat after it boils. I take out three tablespoons of toasted oats, a quarter cup of milk, 13 almonds, 15 raisins, a quarter teaspoon of cinnamon powder and agave syrup. It becomes one full delicious cup of oats; great breakfast, so filling and satisfying.

Bone Health: Barley contains the perfect combination of iron, phosphorous, calcium, magnesium, manganese and zinc, which contribute to building and maintaining bone structure and strength. Consuming two servings in a day helps to enhance the bone health, and one does not need to take calcium supplements.

Heart Health: Barley is rich in fiber, potassium, folate and vitamin B6 content, which support a healthy heart. Barley is an excellent source of fiber, which helps to lower the cholesterol in the blood, thus reducing the risk of heart disease. Barley also contains beta glucan fiber that contributes to lower the cholesterol level. So you have to consume two servings daily to strengthen and protect your heart.

Helps Avoid Cancer: Most of the foods do not contain selenium, which is an important mineral, and it is present in barley. Selenium plays an essential role to strengthen the liver function and helps detoxify some cancer-causing compounds in the body. Selenium also helps prevent inflammation, and tumor growth. Barley grass juice is also very effective to strengthen the body and degenerate cancer cells. 2 Oz of barley grass juice helps assimilate in the blood channel immediately and helps the patient feel less fatigued.

Disables Cancer Cells and Tumor: The fiber in barley also supports heart health. Fiber intake from plant-based foods is also helpful to lower the risk of colon cancer. This high fiber has also been found to stimulate the digestive system, to disable the cancer cells and prevent forming tumors.

Helps Relieve Inflammation: There is a vital and versatile nutrient in barley called Choline, which contributes to sleep, learning, muscle movement, and memory. Choline also helps in the absorption of fat and reduces chronic inflammation.

Helps Get Rid of Constipation: Because of its high fiber content, barley contributes to relieve constipation and promotes natural bowel movement. It is a wise step to consume high fiber food every day to stay regular and healthy. Constipated people always feel sluggish, but your daily consumption of high fiber diet will stimulate your metabolism and make you feel light and fresh.

Obesity and Weight Management: To lose weight and for weight management, in both cases, you need to consume a lot of high fiber foods. Consuming a proper fiber intake is commonly recognized as an important factor in weight loss. Your metabolism has to function properly. Otherwise, you will not see any gain. Diet with fiber helps to satiate your pallet, making you feel fuller for a longer period, thus you consume fewer calories.

Here is my little personal story: I try and test many things on me to see if they work! In 2012, my husband and I decided not to consume dairy products due to GMO contents and strictly eat home-made food. With the consent of my doctor, I started using oats for breakfast, salty pancakes with cooked vegetables or a bowl of cooked beans or lentils. We tried and created new recipes and noticed we were eating more fruits and vegetables. After six week, my husband lost 5 pounds, and I lost 4 pounds in the period of six weeks. So this is the gain when we consume a lot of fiber food.

Beans

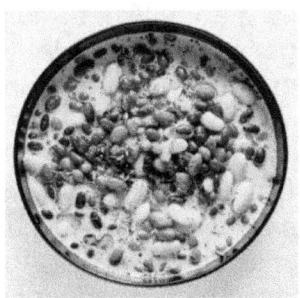

Beans are excellent food that contains protein and fiber and are called a powerhouse of nutrients with antioxidants, vitamins and minerals such folate, phosphorous, potassium, magnesium, manganese, and copper. Beans are known for the good carbs, to provide protein and nutrients and these seeds come under the category of a plant-based food. Beans go great with vegetables.

Help Lose Weight: Because seeds are considered good carbs and metabolized more slowly than other complex carbs, they satiate your pallet thus feeling full without being excessively high in calories. Also, you do not munch on junk food all day, and there is a possibility you may lose some weight.

Nutrient-Rich: Beans are filled with a powerhouse of nutrients including antioxidants, and vitamins and minerals, such as copper, folate, iron, zinc, magnesium, manganese, phosphorous, and potassium. These beans also contain a fair amount of protein, high fiber, and good carbs. The Dietary Guidelines for Americans say that most of us are not consuming enough of these nutrients, and further, they guide us to absorb these powerful nutrients to enhance and maintain our health. Beans by themselves are a complete meal. You can pick kidney beans, black-eyed peas, garbanzo beans, soy beans, pinto beans, mung beans, navy beans or black beans. Add them to your salad plate with the dressing of your choice and enjoy a delicious meal.

Helps Heart Health: Beans are heart healthy food and contain an abundance of soluble fiber, which helps lower cholesterol and triglyceride numbers. If you soak them overnight, then these beans produce less gas and tend to soften faster. I always boil and cook beans at home because canned beans carry a lot of salt and preservatives. If you buy canned beans, then do not forget to rinse them properly to eliminate the sodium content.

Beans Are Low In Fat: Most of the beans contain about 2 to 3 percent fat and carry no cholesterol. We Indians eat beans and lentils every day either at lunch or dinner. Processed or canned beans contain a lot of sodium and salt, but you may wash them before you consume. It is wise to read the label always when you buy any canned food to know what else it contains. I soak them overnight and cook them in a pressure cooker; it takes a little time to prepare. It is high in taste and low on waist. I call it a pure, healthy food.

Beans contain Protein: It is important for us to live by The Dietary Guidelines for Americans which tells us to eat more plant protein to stay healthy. Half a cup of beans provides 7 grams of protein and it is full of fiber. Vegetarians, vegans, and individuals like me, who do not eat meat, poultry, or fish can count on beans as a choice. Some individuals love to consume protein powders and tablets to build muscles, but vegetarians can consume soy and kidney beans and also make muscles.

Great to Balance Blood Sugar: Beans come under a low-glycemic index and contain enough complex carbohydrates. They also contain protein. These beans get digested slowly, keep you satisfied and help to keep blood glucose stable. Wheat converts into sugar, but if you use beans, lentils, and other grains, then blood sugar remains stable. Consuming beans and lentils every day helps to stimulate the digestive system, which makes a natural bowel movement and eliminate constipation too.

They Cut Cancer Risk: Beans and lentils contain so much fiber and antioxidants, now scientists have started recommending that adults consume half a cup of beans per day to promote health, and this helps reduce the risk of chronic diseases, like cancer, constipation, and obesity. This exceptional quality in beans is only because of their abundance of fiber and antioxidants.

Remove Constipation: Constipation is the primary cause of most diseases in our body. Beans, packed with fiber, can help to promote regularity by preventing illness. When you eat half a cup of beans daily, you intend to drink more water that contributes to a natural bowel movement. When you eat intelligently adding high-fiber foods such as beans, fruits and vegetables, your metabolism stays stimulated naturally and you feel light and active all the time. The seeds contain natural protein, nutrients, and compounds that body happily absorbs. Beans are also ideal for those individuals who are sensitive to gluten. Some people get gas after consuming beans, so here is a suggestion: soak beans overnight and use a lot of ginger and garlic when you cook.

Inexpensive and Easy To Cook: Beans are available in many forms. You may buy frozen, canned, or dry, and easy to prepare and store. Now bean flour is also available in Indian stores and the Asian markets. I mix bean flour with wheat and corn flour and make fresh chapattis (tortillas). Also, remember, bean cans are inexpensive and are considered a source of protein. Be a little creative and cook beans at home adding salt, turmeric, black pepper and green peppers. Whenever I cook kidney beans and black eye bean curry, my husband, and I eat a large bowl of this delicious bean-curry because it is so good, filling and satisfying.

Beetroot

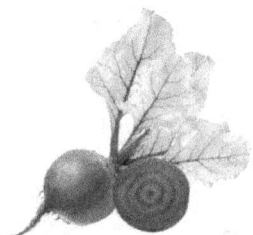

Beetroot commonly known as beets has become popular as a new super food due to recent studies claiming beetroot and its juice can improve physical performance, increase blood flow and lowers blood pressure. I believe in consuming beets in its natural form. While studying Nature Cure, I learned beetroot helps arthritis pain, strengthens the liver, increases the milk in nursing mothers, refreshes brain, and increases blood flow in the body. There are three kinds of beets, red, white and gold; but I have seen only the dark red ones. Only white beets are used to make sugar, which usually helps to sweeten manufactured foods. Red and gold beets, although from the same family, yet are not used to extract sugar.

Obesity: Herbalists and doctors recommend a lot of different fruits and vegetables to help with weight loss and reduce the risk of getting many health conditions. Many studies show and suggest that increasing consumption of plant-based foods such as beetroot decreases the danger of gaining weight. Good carbs keep you feeling full for a longer period of time. It not only helps to control your appetite, it also helps with overall health.

Beauty Enhancing Health: Consumption of beets helps promote a healthy complexion, healthy hair, lowers weight and increases energy. It also increases blood, which is helpful for individuals who are anemic and strengthens the liver and nails. Being high in fiber, it stimulates the digestive system and clears the intestines track. Once you maintain regularity, your face looks calm and relaxed. In India ladies blend beetroot leaves with a little water, a tablespoon of coffee powder and henna. They mix it well and apply this paste on their hair for lustrous and dark hair.

Blood Pressure and Heart Health: I know a folks who drink the juice of one medium beetroot, an apple and a large carrot that makes hardly half a glass, but their acne on the body and face has healed, blood pressure has lowered, and they feel energetic and active. Studies show due to the high nitrate level contained in beetroot could prove to be an inexpensive and effective way to heal heart disorders and blood pressure. Heart patients have to be cautious and consult their doctor before consuming beets because the intake of a lot of beets is not enough for them. Stay only with a quarter of beetroot a day, but you must check with your doctor first.

Dementia: Scientists and researchers at Wake Forest University have found that consuming beetroot juice can improve the intake of oxygen to the brain; that helps to slow the progression of dementia in adults. Per Daniel Kim-Shapiro, Director of Wake Forest's Science Center, in particular areas of the brain, blood flow decrease as we age and the regular intake of beetroot juice leads to rejecting the starting of possible dementia. The blood flow and oxygenation to these areas that are lacking improve with the consumption of beet juice.

Diabetes: Beetroot contains high antioxidant contents, which has been shown to help lower glucose levels and increase insulin for diabetic patients. Because beetroots' sweetness is 100% natural, the body absorbs it faster and contributes to producing energy. Stay only with a quarter beetroot a day.

Digestion and Constipation: Because of its high fiber content, beets help to prevent constipation and promote natural bowel movement for a healthy digestive tract. Adding to your plate of salad or juicing raw beet keeps the digestive system stimulated and healthy. When you maintain regularity, you do not suffer from digestion problems.

Inflammation: Beetroot also contains Choline, which is a crucial and versatile nutrient and helps with insomnia, muscle movement issues, learning and memory. Choline also helps inflammation in the bones thus reducing arthritis pain in the joints.

Exercise and Physical Performance: Beetroot juice has been proven to improve muscle oxygenation during the workout. Due to its nitrate content intake, it has the potential to increase the tolerance and endurance while performing a vigorous exercise. Individuals, who have physical problems such as cardiovascular, respiratory, or metabolic diseases and find their daily activities difficult to perform because of lack of oxygenation. By including beetroot in their diet, they will see improvement.

NOTE: - When you eat beetroot, next day **you will find your bowl movement has a red color**, and this may scare you. It is advisable to consult your doctor before you start eating beetroot.

Berries

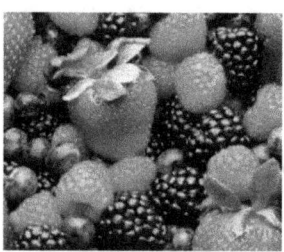

They are little in size, but blueberries, blackberries, boysenberries, raspberries, strawberries, and cranberries are big in antioxidants.

Free radicals that can lead to ailments, can help control the condition with the consumption of these berries. Consuming a diet rich in antioxidants can always help improve human health, protect the skin and hair, and prevent many physical disorders. Most fruits and vegetables contain antioxidants, so including nutrient-rich berries in your diet will ensure you get the antioxidants your body needs. If you do not want to be sick, consume any medicine, or you desire to stay heart healthy, then best practice is to plan a diet rich in nutrients, antioxidants, minerals, enzymes, and high fiber.

Let us see what the berries say: They hold several potent antioxidants that include anthocyanins, and vitamin C. Anthocyanins give berries the vibrant color, help reduces inflammation, and may help prevent and reduce arthritis pain. Studies show Anthocyanins and quercetin work together to help slow memory loss. Quercetin can decrease the inflammation of the joints for people with inflammatory conditions like rheumatoid arthritis.

Vitamin C: It is another adamant and powerful antioxidant found in berries. It mostly helps to maintain the health of collagen, which leads to help maintain and store cartilage and increases joint flexibility. Consuming vitamin C - rich berries contributes to promoting a glow on your skin and beautiful, healthy hair. It can reduce the risk of cataracts, macular degeneration, and arthritis if you eat rich in antioxidant foods on daily basis.

High Water Content: These berries are full of juice and contain mostly water, and foods that possess so much water are best for weight loss. Because of their high water content, they fill you up faster, and you are putting fewer calories into your body. These berries contain fiber and folate also. Consuming food rich in fiber helps in weight loss and also leads to lower cholesterol and blood pressure. Folate is a great compound that protects against heart disease and memory loss in matured people. Folate is believed to contribute the production of serotonin, which ultimately can aid to remove depression and improve your mood.

NOTE: - Individuals, who suffer from Irritable Bowel Syndrome, they sometimes experience **discomfort while consuming berries**. Please remember, here we are talking and trying to be healthier and not sick; so please stay away from those berries that are not compatible with your system.

Blueberries, Blackberries, Boysenberries, Cranberries, Raspberries, and Strawberries: Blueberries make a great fruit eat if you are trying to lose weight because they consist of 80% water. They also contain a high level of antioxidants which helps with arthritis, memory loss in matured individuals, and cataracts and many eyesight problems.

Blackberries: Blackberries contain more than 85% water along with a lot of fibers; that makes them an excellent fruit to consume if you want to lose weight; help lower cholesterol, and manage sugar level. These berries are an excellent source of folate, which is a vitamin B and it contributes to maintaining healthy hair and nails. Blackberries also may reduce the risk of heart disease and mood swings. Moreover, blackberries are full of potent antioxidants, which help with arthritis pain and memory loss in matured people, cataracts, and eyesight problems.

Boysenberries: Boysenberries are a cross of raspberries, blackberries, and loganberries, and they look like a giant version of a blackberry. Boysenberries contain anthocyanins, which are potent antioxidants that can help with arthritis and age-related memory loss.

Cranberries: Cranberries contain 85% water with high fiber, but most people do not consume raw because they are too sour and astringent. Instead, cranberries are usually enjoyed in sweetened form, either dried berries or sweet with sugar cranberry sauce. Diabetic patients should try to limit their consumption because these berries are concentrated sources of sugar. Diabetic people should try their best to avoid their intake of sugary sweetened berries. Both fresh and dried cranberries are an excellent source of anthocyanins, anti-inflammatory antioxidants and are helpful with arthritis pain and memory loss.

Raspberries: Raspberries contain more than 85 percent water along with a hefty dose of fiber, which makes them a great fruit to eat if you're trying to lose weight, lower cholesterol, or manage type 2 diabetes. They are also full of potent antioxidants, including vitamin C and anthocyanins, which can help with arthritis, age-related memory loss, cataracts and other eyesight problems, and maintaining healthy skin and hair.

Strawberries: Strawberry holds more than 90 percent water along with a hefty dose of fiber, which makes it a great fruit to eat if you're trying to lose weight, lower cholesterol or manage type 2 diabetes. They are an excellent source of folate, a B vitamin that helps maintain healthy hair and may reduce the risk of cardiovascular disease and mood disorders. Additionally, strawberries are full of potent antioxidants, including vitamin C and anthocyanins, which can help with arthritis, age-related memory loss, cataracts and other eyesight problems, and maintaining healthy skin and hair. IF YOU HAVE THYROID ISSUES, YOU SHOULD STAY AWAY FROM THEM

NOTE: - All berries are a nutritious fruit and if you cannot afford to buy them then buy them when they are on sale. Freeze them, and use whenever you desire.

Bitter Melon

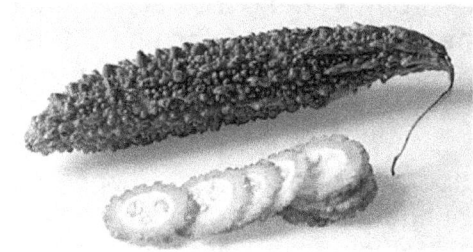

Bitter melon is an excellent vegetable for the body. We call It a blood purifier. I would like to advise all my readers to eat this vegetable on a daily basis. It helps cure diabetes and cleanses the digestive system. In India, diabetic patients are treated with its powder and juice. It is bitter and we call it Karela. I cook it with ghee, lots of onions, tomatoes, and ginger, and it is delightful. In spite of its bitterness, people consume it raw because it helps relieve many skin disorders. It is a unique vegetable, and we use as food and medicine. It all depends on what you want to put in your body. Regular consumption of this plant contributes to glowing skin and a youthful body because it cleanses the blood. It contains Vitamin C, which is a potent antioxidant and can fight and eliminate harmful free radicals. It also aids in preventing fine lines by slowing down the aging process and protects our skin from damage from the sun's UV rays.

It purifies our blood, an excellent agent for people having diabetes and improves constipation and hemorrhoids. It is also helpful in healing skin disorders, possesses Vitamins B and Vitamin C and is a rich source of minerals such as iron, phosphorous, and calcium. I try my best to include this vegetable in our food once a week. In fact, it is one of our favorite plant food, I cook bharvan karela, cut into 1/2 an inch wide rings and sautéed. I cook bitter melon in a variety of recipes, and it comes out delicious. (You may consult my book "Scrumptious Meals from India, Volume 3"). You can add onions, tomatoes, and bell peppers to make this dish a delicious one.

Healing Qualities Overall: Bitter melon helps in controlling blood flow and clotting, aiding wounds in healing faster, thus preventing further infections. Remember; unpleasant things have incredible benefits. It is high in beneficial polyphenols that boost energy and metabolism.

Promotes Anti-Ageing: The healing properties which are present in bitter melon can help slow down the aging process. The free radicals in this vegetables are also very useful for purifying the blood and keeping us healthy, young and vibrant.

Promote Longevity: Bitter melon is an excellent home remedy for longevity. It is very beneficial for skin and health. It is full of nutrients and antioxidants that purify the blood, and when you have no disease in your body, you are going to live long naturally. When patients get its juice to drink in Nature Cure organizations the Ayurvedic practitioners tell them, "Drink the whole thing if you want to live long."

Hair Health: You can use it in many different ways to enhance the health of your hair. You can mix a quarter cup of fresh bitter melon juice with yogurt; apply on your hair and leave it on for 20 minutes. Wash it off and enjoy natural shiny and beautiful hair. Repeat this process twice a week; it will promote the removal of dandruff, repair split ends, and moisturize dry scalp and even new hair growth. If you have long thick hair, then you may make more of this mixture. Bitter melon juice aids in reducing the natural falling out of the hair. Once a week you can add a teaspoon of sugar or honey in its juice and massage on the roots to get better results. If you have thick, and unruly hair, apply two spoons of its water, and that will help you manage your hair easily. You may also use its juice on the roots once a week to reduce gray hair growth.

Respiratory Disorders: It is common in India to witness people boil its fresh pods and drink the water to get relief from respiratory disorders or asthma. People believe it is an excellent remedy for curing respiratory problems such as breathing problems and asthma, the common cold and cough. One may also try its paste made with its delicate leaves mixed with sweet basil (Tulsi) paste and consume it with a little honey each morning to get positive results.

Liver Tonic: Patients with liver conditions also drink 5 oz. of bitter melon juice daily to get rid of liver problems. You may experience positive results after consuming it continuously for one week.

Immune System: Some people boil bitter melon leaves in water and eat and drink its water every day to fight against infections. It also helps cleanse the digestive system and build your immunity.

Acne: Regular consumption of bitter melon can get rid of acne, blemishes, and skin disorders. It is beneficial in treating blood disorders like itching, blood boils, fungal diseases, scabies, psoriasis, and ringworm. Consume the juice of a bitter melon mixed with lemon on an empty stomach daily for three months or till you get the desired results.

Diabetes: Bitter melon juice is very beneficial for diabetic patients. In India, Ayurvedic practitioners give its water and powder to cure diabetes. They also give this vegetable to their diabetic patients to eat every day as it contains potent chemicals and antioxidant compounds that safeguard the food that does not convert into sugar. Some of its elements are very high, and they work like insulin in assisting the decrease the blood sugar level. Indian and Chinese herbalists have been using this plant for centuries and treating their patients for so many physical conditions.

Heart Health: Bitter melon is an excellent vegetable for the heart in several ways. It contributes to reducing the harmful cholesterol that accumulates in the arteries and aids in reducing the chances of heart attacks. Also, it assists in lowering the blood sugar level which helps in maintaining a good healthy heart.

Cancer: Bitter melon can degenerate the cancer cells and assist in preventing cancer cells from multiplying.

Weight Loss: Bitter melon includes high antioxidants and fiber that contribute in flushing out your system. It carries 80-85% water which is a filling agent and the known universal suppressant of hunger. This vegetable stimulates your metabolism and digestive systems, thus helping you lose weight faster. It is low in calories and has little fat. You may consume a significant amount and still lose some weight.

Skin Infections: This unique vegetable benefits the treatment of skin infections and skin diseases such as eczema, psoriasis, itches, and rashes. The regular consumption of bitter melon juice improves psoriasis and fungal infections like ringworm. It also contributes to keeping your skin glowing and free from blemishes. If one starts eating healthy from childhood, then there is no chance of acne or blemishes as its benefits purify the blood.

Constipation: This plant helps in easy digestion as it includes high fiber properties. After its consumption food is digested and waste is pushed out of the body which helps with indigestion and constipation problems.

Kidney and Bladder stones: This vegetable assists in maintaining a healthy gallbladder and liver. Regular consumption of bitter melons helps dissolve the kidney rocks and passes them through the urinary tract in small pieces. It also enhances kidney health and better functioning of the kidneys.

Bottle Gourd

Bottle gourd is not very popular here in the USA, but in India it is not only famous but #1 favorite vegetable to everyone. We call it lauki or ghiya. Everyone probably knows this food in India for its delicious preparations in a large variety. Though its taste is a little bitter, which after cooking you will not feel, yet it is highly nutritional in value, and we cannot ignore that. In fact, Ayurvedic practitioners and Natural Cure therapists recommend the consumption of this bottle gourd to treat various conditions. Consuming bottle gourd juice has many health benefits. This green vegetable is full of nutrients, vitamins, enzymes, minerals and water. Making this an essential part of your food intake. Bottle gourd is good to pacify liver inflammation, healthy digestion, and premature graying of the hair.

Diarrhea: If you are suffering from diarrhea, take bottle gourd juice with a pinch of sea salt two to three times a day, and loose stools will stop. It works to maintain electrolyte balance in the body and is an excellent remedy for Individuals who have diarrhea.

Constipation: The consumption of bottle gourd is very beneficial for those, who suffer from constipation because it is high in fiber and helps clear the food trapped in the colon. Moreover, its juice helps in the treatment of acidity as it is an alkaline food. The high fiber and the minerals which appear in it contributes healthy digestion and fights flatulence and constipation.

Weight Loss: Bottle gourd juice is widely used for weight loss and to lower the bad cholesterol for the obese. In India, bottle gourd juice is available on each corner and is inexpensive so that everyone can take advantage of this simple vegetable to be fit and be beautiful. It is highly popular for weight loss. My cousin, who is a judge, lives in India, sent me an email saying, "I am not allowed to eat fried food. I am on a diet plan of chapatti with zucchini and bottle gourd, and I have lost 22 pounds." Wow! It sounds great.

Kidneys: Ayurvedic practitioners recommend bottle gourd juice to individuals, who suffer from kidney-related problems. It aids to reduce the inflammation in the kidneys. It enhances the health of the kidneys so that they can function well. Like cranberries, bottle gourd supports the urinary system of the body and aids from a burning sensation. It also helps reduce the chance of urinary infection because it is alkalizing and has a diuretic effect.

Lowers High Blood Pressure: Bottle gourd is highly famous for the reduction of high blood pressure and helps keep the heart healthy. In India, people cook this vegetable very often.

Hair: As per Ancient Ayurveda, bottle gourd can prevent prematurely the graying of hair. You need to drink a fresh bottle of gourd juice in the morning possibly on an empty stomach each day.

Sleep: If someone has an insomnia condition, then eat the bottle gourd cooked with two teaspoons of sesame oil. When we mix one teaspoon of sesame oil with bottle gourd juice, it also contributes to curing problems of sleep disorder.

Broccoli

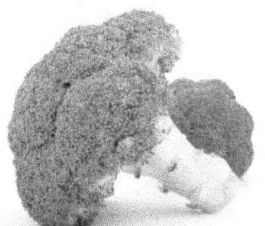

We all know the great benefits of broccoli and its many rich nutrients. It contains the most nutritional compounds. It has vitamins and disease-fighting chemicals. Here are some of the benefits of broccoli:

Helps Cancer Prevention: Broccoli contains immune boosting properties similar to vegetables such as cauliflower, cabbage, kale and Brussels sprouts. Medical professionals always recommend these kinds of plant foods to their cancer patients. Herbalists use broccoli for prevention of disease.

Helps Cholesterol Reduction: Broccoli contains high fiber that helps lower cholesterol, and this is one of the healthiest foods in the whole world.

Powerful antioxidant: Broccoli also is an excellent source of vitamin C, and some people consider it a powerhouse of antioxidants. The consumption of potent antioxidants increases the digestion, nutrients, and the value of the food. Vegetables should be an essential staple for the humans.

Help Reduce Inflammation: Broccoli helps to lower the inflammatory condition in the body. The high fiber it contains is helpful to cleanse the digestive system and enhance our health.

Helps Strengthen Bones: Broccoli contains high levels of Vitamin K and Calcium and these both are healthy compounds, which are essential to strength human bones. Regularly eating broccoli helps make bones strong and healthy. Vitamin K and calcium are not only necessary for bone health, but it is essential for the prevention of osteoporosis.

Heart Health: Broccoli holds the anti-inflammatory properties, which can help to prevent some of the damage caused by inflammatory conditions. In Nature Cure, we believe these kinds of vegetables can even help reverse the damage also. One must plan a healthy diet plan to enhance one's health condition.

Diet Aid: Broccoli is a good carb and is rich in fiber that helps in digestion, prevents constipation, maintains low blood sugar, and curbs overeating. When you consume these kinds of vegetables every day, you do not have to work hard to lose weight, and you will notice your body fat is melting naturally and quickly. Additionally, a cup of broccoli has as much protein as a cup of rice or corn with half the calories.

Note: - Broccoli and all the cruciferous vegetables that contain high contents of antioxidants, **interrupt the benefits of your medicines like Coumadin or Warfarin (for blood thinning)** if consumed in a large quantity daily. You must consult your physician before you start planning to eat these vegetables.

Cabbage

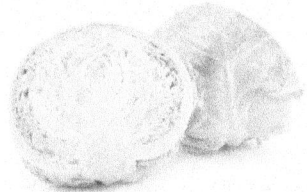

When buying groceries, pick up a cabbage that is heavy for its size and make sure the leaves are firm and tight as the loose leaves indicate an older piece. You can store cabbage in the refrigerator for two to three weeks. You may consume cabbage raw, roasted, steamed, boiled, or sautéed. When you overcook cabbage, then you can smell its sulfurous odor but remember, overcooked vegetable lose their nutrients and benefits.

Consuming fruits and vegetables of all kinds have always been helpful in reducing the risk of many adverse health problems. The studies suggest increasing the consumption of plant foods like cabbage, decreases the likelihood of diabetes, obesity, heart conditions and other diseases. It is the one top vegetable that promotes a healthy body, bright complexion, increased energy, and overall lowers the weight.

Helps Protect from radiation therapy: Cabbage contains a compound known as cruciferous that is also available in some other vegetables such as cauliflower and broccoli. This content has been shown to protect against the horrible effects of radiation therapy. This useful compound has protective effects against cancer, and also shows there is hope for using it as a shield to protect healthy tissues during cancer treatment in the coming future.

Helps Prevent Cancer: Researchers say the sulfur-containing compound that gives cruciferous vegetables a different kind of taste also gives them the cancer-fighting power. More studies are on the way for sulforaphane compound and scientists are hoping that this compound will help to disable the cancer bacteria. Another natural chemical in cabbage, parsley, celery, and other plants known as apigenin has been discovered which assists with cancer. It may also be utilized as a potential compound to use for safe treatment for cancer in the future.

Red cabbage is believed to be the powerhouse of antioxidant anthocyanin, the same compound that gives others it's red and purple-hued fruits and vegetables their vibrant colors. Anthocyanins have been shown to slow cancer cells, kill already formed cancer cells and helps stop the formation of new tumor growth. Red cabbage tends to contain more of these compounds than green cabbage.

Improves Heart health: The powerful anthocyanin in red cabbage, which helps protect against cancer, has also proved to help suppress inflammation that may lead to the heart disease. The American Journal of Clinical Nutrition published a report about the intake of flavonoid-rich foods that can contribute to lower the risk of death from heart disease and stated even small portions of flavonoid-rich foods consumed on a daily basis, may be beneficial. Another high polyphenol content in cabbage can also help reduce the risk of heart disease and reduce the blood pressure.

Regulates immune system and indigestion: A simple method to consume cabbage is by adding it to your salads. In Nature Cure, eating raw cabbage is like consuming probiotic, which is considered one of the best things you can do easily for your immune and digestive systems. Cabbage contains fiber and water that helps to prevent constipation and maintain a healthy digestive system. Consuming an adequate portion of fiber every day, promotes regularity and natural bowel movement. Normal metabolism gives you a feeling of wellness and being healthy. New studies are proving that the diet rich in fiber may play a huge role in regulating the immune system and inflammation thus decreasing the risk of inflammation-related problems such as heart disease, obesity, diabetes, and even cancer.

Carrots

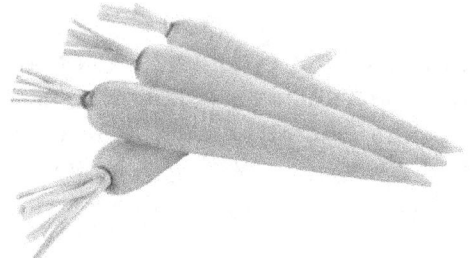

Helps Improve vision: We all know carrots are great for the eyes. Now doctors recommend consuming fresh carrots as they are rich in beta-carotene, which converts into vitamin A in the liver. Vitamin A is essential for our eyes and helps improve our vision and heals the night time blindness. It has also been shown to protect against macular degeneration and slows cataracts to form. People who consume carrots or beta-carotene on a daily basis may experience a lower risk of macular degeneration.

Helps prevent cancer: Carrots reduce the risk of cancer. Besides beta-carotene, researchers have just discovered new and efficient anticancer properties in the carrots. They believe that carrots can help lessen the likelihood of breast cancer, lung cancer, and colon cancer if we consume carrots or carrot juice regularly.

It is Anti-Aging: Beta-carotene works as an antioxidant to damaged cells; that helps slow down the aging of cells. It also helps the metabolism that ultimately brings strength. Carrots help to sharpen memory and also give a little weight to the people, who have poor health if a large glass of juice consumed regularly.

Promotes Healthier Body skin: Carrots of full of vitamin A and antioxidants that protect the skin against sun damage. Deficiencies of vitamin A and antioxidant food make the skin, hair and nails look dry and rough. It repairs your skin and keeps it firm. Vitamin A helps prevent premature wrinkling, acne, dry skin, discoloration, pigmentation, and blemishes. Munching on raw carrots not only helps your gums and teeth but also brings a glow on your face.

Helps prevent infections: In Nature Cure carrots play a significant role. In India, people with all kinds of disorders, are treated with natural foods like fruits, vegetables, and sprouts. They consume carrot juice, steamed carrots, carrot jam and carrot salads. Herbalists very well know the high qualities of carrots to prevent infections. These are also used on cuts – boiled and mashed or shredded raw.

Promotes healthier Facial skin: Carrots are seasonal but these days they are available throughout the year and as an inexpensive food, you can eat them raw, steamed, sautéed, juiced or cooked with any other ingredients like pasta, bean, vegetables or salads. You can make a convenient facial mask also to soften and radiate your facial skin by mixing carrot paste with a teaspoon of honey and juice of half a teaspoon of lemon.

Prevents heart disease and stroke: Carrots contain not only beta-carotene but also lutein and alpha-carotene that are an essential nutrient to enhance human health, especially eyes health. Harvard University study shows, individuals, who consumed more than six carrots a week, have fewer chances to suffer from a stroke than those, who ate fewer carrots in a month. Diets with high nutrients help to lower the risk of heart disease and prevent a stroke.

Cleanses the body: Vitamin A helps the liver in flushing out the toxins from the. body. The high fibers, which carrots contain help clean out the colon and make a smooth bowel movement. Regular consumption of carrots detoxifies the digestive system. When I was studying in beauty college, my lunch was only carrots five days a week for six months as I had no time to eat lunch. I packed cut up carrots in a zip-log bag at night, took them to work next day and while going from my job to beauty college at 12:00 noon I ate carrots for my lunch when I was on the wheels. I realized I did not gain any weight, was never sick during that period and felt energized and healthier. Sometimes, my boss came and grabbed a couple of pieces of carrots saying, "Gee, I have to go to a conference, this will cleanse my mouth and freshen up my breath."

Protects teeth and gums: Carrots clean our teeth and mouth and scrape off the plaque and food particles just like a toothbrush and the toothpaste. Chewing carrots stimulate gums due to its crunchy nature. It triggers more saliva, that being alkaline, balances the acid-forming and cavity-forming bacteria. Carrots also contain minerals that prevent tooth damage.

NOTE: - Now you do not need a vitamin pill. Just add crunchy orange powerful carrots in your life; you will get natural vitamin A with other powerful health benefits including cancer prevention, beautiful skin, and anti-aging too. Try to get maximum healthy benefits from this amazing vegetable.

Cauliflower

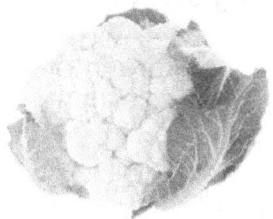

Cauliflower contains a high level of the sulfur compound. It is known to support the liver's ability to neutralize the toxins. Most of the vegetables of this family also have the capacity to help prevent different cancers.

Source of Calcium: Cauliflower is a source of calcium that has several benefits. Calcium contributes to strengthening our bones and teeth along with the ability to thicken our hair. It is important to consume half a cup of this vegetable, raw, steamed or sautéed at least four days a week for healthy bones.

Source of Rich Minerals: Cauliflower contains zinc, manganese, phosphorus, magnesium and also selenium and sodium.

Zinc helps in producing new cells and also heals wounds.

Magnesium helps the parathyroid gland that produces hormones to strength the bone to function normally.

Phosphorus contributes to strengthening the bones.

Selenium helps the immune system to alleviate its functions.

Sodium helps balance the fluids in the whole body.

Manganese helps in producing and activating the enzymes.

Helps Promote Heart Health: Cauliflower is a heart healthy vegetable, helps in maintaining the heart health and the cardiovascular system.

Helps Lower Cholesterol: Cauliflower contains nutritional benefits, include being rich in fiber. Food rich in fiber helps in lowering your Cholesterol levels.

Supports Healthy Immune System: Cauliflower contains antioxidants, which has numerous benefits. They work as anti-inflammatory agents, and they help build a healthy immune system.

Development of Fetus: Cauliflower is rich in folate and helps women during pregnancy. Because of its high content of folate and vitamins such as vitamin A and vitamin B, it helps in growing the body cells. Cauliflower eventually helps in the proper development of the fetus in the womb. Additionally, cauliflower is also an excellent source of vitamin C, which again is beneficial for the pregnant women. In Nature Cure, we recommend pregnant women to consume at least one cup of cauliflower every day. They may eat raw, steamed or sautéed, the kind of their choice.

Help Reduce Cancer Risk: Cauliflower helps in reducing the likelihood of cancer. The cruciferous family of vegetables like cauliflower, broccoli, kale and squash aid to decrease the risk of diseases like breast cancer, bladder cancer, and lung cancer.

In India, people with different kinds of cancers are treated with cruciferous vegetables` juices, and dishes like steamed, boiled, sautéed and cooked with ginger and garlic.

Helps Promote Weight Loss: Cauliflower helps to lose weight if consumed every day. Cauliflower contains vitamin C that is the main element to help melt fat. It also contains folate that again helps to promote lose weight. One cup of cauliflower is a good portion to consume. It contains approximately 30 calories; it has no starch, and one can consume as much as one wants.

Helps Cleanse the Body System: The vitamin C and the fiber, cauliflower contains helps the body to activate enzymes in the liver that helps in detoxifying body organs thus protecting the system from bacteria. It is full of lots of minerals that are essential for the body to keep us healthy and fit.

How Cauliflower Rejuvenates Skin: Cauliflower is full of beneficial properties that help us to stay healthy and beautiful. The best benefit of consuming cauliflower is it contributes to rejuvenate your skin.

As Cauliflower contains potent antioxidants such as vitamin C, folate, and fiber, it is an excellent vegetable to stimulate metabolism that works as anti-aging agents for the skin. These nutrients help to bring more oxygen in the blood which enhances our health and brings a glow on the face. Remember when you consume these kinds of vegetables with the abundance of nutrients, you detoxify your body on daily basis. Just start bringing vegetables and fruits in your life to look and feel younger, healthy and ageless.

Helps Boost Vitamin K Content: If you have a deficiency of Vitamin K in your body, then cauliflower is the one to boost it in your system. You can increase the intake of cauliflower with your meals to boost Vitamin k as it plays the key role to develop the bone cells. **There can be an increased amount of bleeding if a wound or injury occurs when your body does not have enough vitamin K**. You must consult your doctor before you increase the intake of vitamin K because sometimes it interrupts with your blood thinning medicine.

Celery

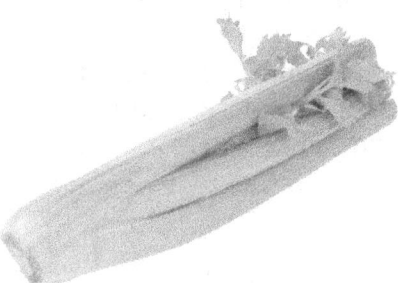

Celery contains an endless list of health benefits, and I am sure you will also start liking it when you read to know its functional benefits. Before you start any food plan, select more vegetables, which have the same effect so that you can make a large plate with salads every day.

Helps You In Stress: Celery is an excellent food for stress-relief. It contains the precious minerals such as magnesium and the essential oil in it that soothes the nervous system. You need one celery stalk as a snack that helps calm your mind and sleep better.

Helps Lose Weight: Celery will be an excellent choice if you want to lose pounds. One large celery stalk contains only ten calories. Regularly consuming celery in your salads, soups, and stir-fries or even with peanut butter will help you reach your goal.

Helps Regulate Body Balance: Celery comes under the category of alkaline food that helps regulates the body's alkaline balance, thus contributes to protecting from indigestion and acidity.

Helps The Digestion: Celery is full of water, contains a high level of insoluble fiber that promotes natural bowel movement. It contains "good" salts. Yes, celery does contain sodium, but it is not the same thing as table salt. The salt in celery is organic, natural and essential for your health.

Helps Your Eyes: One large stalk of celery can give you up to 10 percent of Vitamin A, and that is the daily dose what a human body needs. Vitamin A is an important nutrient that enhances eyes health as well as protects the eyes and prevents age-related deterioration of vision.

Helps Reduces Cholesterol: Researchers believe celery also includes a component that helps reduce bad cholesterol (LDL) and also It is responsible for giving its flavor and scent to this vegetable. One can eat two stalks of celery a day to reduce bad cholesterol.

Helps Reduce Inflammation: Regular consumption of celery can help individuals suffering from joint pains, asthma, lung infections, or acne by reducing the inflammation in the joints and intestines.

Pressure Helps Lower The Blood: Celery contains an active and beneficial compound that has already helped in boosting circulatory health. Consuming raw, whole celery reduces high blood pressure.

Helps Boost Youthfulness: Celery can also boost up your sex life. Dr. Alan R. Hirsch, Director of the Smell and Taste Treatment and Research Foundation, says that two particular kinds of hormones are present in celery that help men's vigor and boost the sex lives. Celery only releases those hormones when they chew on the celery stalks.

Celery Helps Avoid Cancer: A powerful flavonoid in the celery is present that can help stop the growth of cancer bacteria, especially in the pancreas. Other studies advise the regular consumption of celery may help delay the formation of breast cancer cells.

NOTE: - As a rule of thumb select celery that is fresh and crisp. The darker the color, the stronger the flavor. It is better to eat fresh chopped celery than cut into pieces and store in the refrigerator. Celery has diuretic and cleansing properties; it is advisable not to consume celery if you have diarrhea.

Cilantro

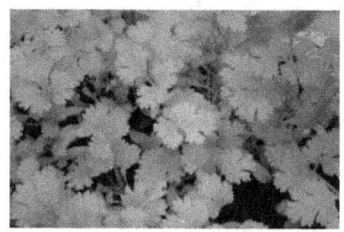

Cilantro is a blessing for humanity. It is rich in crucial vitamins and antioxidants such as beta-carotene, folate, and vitamin C that holds a fresh and an aromatic flavor. Cilantro offers us a variety of great health benefits.

Heart Health: Cilantro is a herb and it is cholesterol free. It is rich in antioxidants, vitamins, essential oils, and dietary fiber that help to lower bad cholesterol (LDL) and increase good cholesterol (HDL). Thus, helping the patients with a heart condition and also helps dissolve cholesterol build up in the arteries.

Strengthens Kidney: Cilantro is excellent for kidney problems. It strengthens the kidney and helps make the toxins push out of the body. It is a proven fact. It also helps regulate the kidney function.

Helps Lower Blood Pressure: Cilantro not only lowers cholesterol but also contributes to reducing hypertension. This herb also makes little easy on the heart. The herb contains an excellent source of calcium, potassium, magnesium, manganese and iron. Its high potassium and low sodium level also help control blood pressure and heart rate.

Digestive Aid: Cilantro leaves and stems give relief in indigestion problems as well as sick feelings. They also hold antioxidant benefits that help to promote the liver function. This herb includes fiber too, which helps stimulate the digestive system.

Excessive Heavy Metal Detoxifier: In India, people believe cilantro is a wonderful detoxifier. Herbalists claim it can remove excessive metal consumption from the human body that enter through the variety of foods. This metallic intake mostly enters the body through consumption of non-organic food, drinking unfiltered water, using hairspray, smoking, cooking food wrapped in aluminum foil, or consuming over the counter drugs. These sources can create serious health problems and various diseases.

Helps Sleep Well: Cilantro is a favorite herb with calming effects. It can contribute to improving the quality of your sleep as it is a calming herb, thus reducing anxiety and stress.

Anti-diabetic Properties: Since cilantro has high potassium and low sodium it has been very useful for diabetic patients. It can help in regulating and keeping their blood sugar stable. Cilantro also contributes to lower the cholesterol and blood sugar if regularly consumed.

Anti-inflammatory Effects: Cilantro contains a high level of anti-inflammatory capacities which helps eliminate inflammatory conditions like arthritis and reduce minor swelling. It is a high powered herb and helps prevent many physical problems.

Helps Sooth Hemorrhoids: Cilantro is popular for its healing properties. If one bunch of cilantro, one pack of curry leaves, and one bunch of sweet basil are combined and ground to a paste, then consume one spoonful of it first thing in the morning with a cup of water every day. You may store the rest of the mix in the refrigerator for future use. If consumed for a longer period, it helps to hang nails in hemorrhoids, decreases pain, and eventually stops the bleeding. In India, I know a lady, who had a severe problem of hemorrhoids, consumed this for a couple of years and noticed her hemorrhoids cured long back also her hair became thick and lustrous.

Helps Heal Stress And Anxiety: Due to its calming and muscle relaxing qualities, cilantro helps in soothing the nerves, thus relieving from anxiety. It also contributes to reducing the harmful effects of stress because of its cleansing capacity. Drinking cilantro juice combined with two celery sticks and a cucumber with one green apple at the end of the day, especially after work, is so refreshing for replenishing your body with vitamins B to help sooth your mind and body. You feel de-stressed and also, you lose weight if you regularly consume it.

Coconut Oil

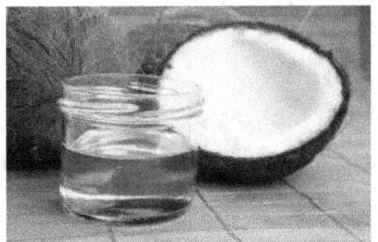

The experts have phased out all the saturated oils from our lives and have replaced it with 'healthy vegetable and seed oils.' Why the experts are not ready to understand that it is not the fat that gives us diseases or heart attack, but it is the bad fat that hurts us and makes us sick. What makes us sick is, the fried food we all love and eat all the time. The packaged foods that the big companies are manufacturing with lots of low grade and cheap oils and add lots of unwanted contents such as salt, sugar, chemicals as preservatives to make their foods delicious, increased shelf life and were minting money. We need to understand saturated fats and oils are essential for cell function and growth. Our body needs fat for energy and strength for our day-to-day life.

I use a little butter every day but I never use margarine. I swirl organic coconut oil on top of my cooked meals but never use it while cooking, meaning I do not heat it. My husband and I rarely eat out. When I was studying Nature Cure my teachers emphasized eating fat; it has to be pure and in small quantities. Furthermore, my instructors told me even if I want to lose weight, fats are necessary for the proper functioning of the body.

Coconut oil is in vogue. In India people use coconut oil a lot. In South India, coconut grows in abundance and mostly residents on the seaside are the biggest users of it in their day-to-day life. The surprising thing is that most of the population in the south is thin.

People of Thailand use coconut oil in abundance and most of the people are known to be thin with little to no disease. Over 1/3 of the world's population depends on coconut for food and its oil. It's time to consider incorporating coconut oil into your daily diet and get this packed powerhouse nutrient into your lifestyle. Amongst the oils in day-to-day use, Coconut oil stands like a shining star for its innumerable valid values for the consumer.

Coconut helps reduce inflammation: People believe coconut oil works as an anti-inflammatory agent. The high level of antioxidants appears in coconut oil reduces inflammation and heals arthritis pain effectively. The fatty acids (Lauric Acid) in coconut oil can reduce the inflammation internally and externally; thus to moisturize and make them an excellent solution for all types of skin conditions.

Cancer: People call coconut 'A Super Food' and believe it directly protects the liver from damage. Its water contributes to hydrate and support the healing process. Coconut oil can fight cancer because while digesting, it produces ketones and tumor cells are unable to contact the energy in ketones and they need glucose to function. People believe a particular diet on ketones can be a possible way to help cancer patients recover and feel better. Herbalists also tell us if coconut oil is introduced to the cancer patients before they get the chemical into the body, it can prevent cancer from developing further.

Alzheimer Disease: Latest research shows that the brain creates insulin and works on it to process the glucose and power brain cells. When an individual loses the ability to produce insulin that is the time when Alzheimer disease starts. The ketones from coconut oil can generate an alternate source of energy for the repair of the brain to work properly.

Heart Disease and High Blood Pressure: Coconut oil is highly equipped with natural saturated fats that contribute to increasing the healthy cholesterol in the body, and we call it HDL. Moreover, coconut oil helps to convert the "bad" cholesterol (LDL) into good cholesterols. When the healthy cholesterol increases in our body, it promotes heart health and lowers the risk of heart disease. Because it includes very essential contents with its anti-inflammatory and anti-oxidant compounds, coconut oil is very helpful to human health.

Kidney and UTI Problem: Coconut oil is full of beneficial compounds, can improve and heal urinary (UTI) and kidney infections. The essential contents it possesses, act as a natural antibiotic by degenerating the bacteria and killing them. Also, the researchers say coconut water also contributes to hydrate and maintain the healing process. Medical professionals are now even injecting the coconut water to cleanse out the kidney stones. Coconut is a super powerful food!

Boost Immune System: Coconut, being antiviral, anti-fungal, and antibacterial, coconut oil is a potent and powerful agent to fight bacteria in the body. Coconut oil includes Lauric Acid, which is a well-known fact that reduces Candida, fights bacteria, and generates an aggressive environment for viruses. At present many diseases are coming up by the overgrowing of bad bacteria, parasites, viruses, and fungus in the body. Ayurvedic practitioners suggest to take a tablespoon of coconut three times a day when one is sick; possessing a natural fuel source, it disables the bacteria to attach your body cell.

Boost Brain Power & Energy: Coconut oil improves the memory problems in the matured people. While regularly consuming this fatty acid, older individuals feel improved memory and ability to function better in life. It is easy to digest, increases your metabolism, and you feel boosted energy. When you buy coconut oil, select the organic one or look for a quality non-processed coconut oil, so that the beneficial compounds can fuel the brain cells more efficiently. It also benefits the liver directly, which eventually converts into energy.

Digestion & Reduce Stomach Ulcer: As we know, coconut oil is an all-rounder and can contribute to improving bacteria and health by just destroying harmful bacteria which makes us sick. When the bacteria are killed or pushed out of the body, it improves the digestion. It also contributes the body to absorb fat-soluble vitamins, magnesium, and calcium. Coconut also improves digestion as it helps the body to absorb fat-soluble vitamins, calcium, and magnesium. If we take Omega-3 fatty acids with coconut oil, its beneficial effects are doubled as per my Nature Cure teacher.

Skin: Now big companies are manufacturing several products with coconut oil, and even the saloons are using it. It is an excellent moisturizer, face cleanser, and sunscreen, and it can help treat many skin problems. The fatty acids (Lauric Acid) in coconut oil reduce inflammation internally and from the skin and promote to moisturize and to make them an excellent solution for infected skin disease. Herbal Therapists believe, it can help to eliminate dandruff, psoriasis, burns, eczema and rash. Moreover, it protects our skin and is full of many antioxidants that promote healing the sore skin.

Prevent Gum Disease And Strengthen Teeth: If you want healthy gums and strong teeth, you may start 'oil pulling' every day in the morning. You swish one tablespoon of coconut oil in your mouth for 20 minutes. (First do a little research about oil pulling and learn the details, only then you should begin). It is not new; people have been doing 'oil pulling' for centuries as a method of cleansing the mouth of bacteria and help heal their tooth problems, because there were no dentists at that time. It is one of the most effective oils for oil pulling due to its high concentration of antibacterial contents. Moving bacteria in the mouth gets washed out by swishing the oil. Removing oral bacteria regularly by oil pulling contributes to reducing your risk of periodontal disease. In my family, my husband, all my daughters and I, regularly do oil pulling and my daughter Seema always brushes her teeth with coconut oil after she drinks coffee; she enjoys beautiful white teeth. Salute to the coconut!

Prevent Osteoporosis: Coconut oil is full with a high level of antioxidants that help fight the free radicals. Ayurvedic practitioners believe it is a leading natural treatment for osteoporosis. It increases calcium absorption in the digestive system. Coconut oil contributes to increasing bone construction and volume and safeguards bone loss due to osteoporosis. Do not cook food with it or burn to fry. Take it in its natural form or the positive results.

Lose Weight: Researchers have done a lot of study on coconut oil, but most of them were on animals. In South India people have used this oil for centuries and in those States, a less number of fat people and diseases prevail. In Thailand people live on coconut oil and there are not too many obese as we have in our country, the USA. Its ability to encourage you to get rid of your extra weight. Because of the energy generating abilities of coconut oil, there is no wonder it is beneficial in shedding some pounds. It promotes to burn fat, suppresses appetite, and you do not like to munch the whole day. I believe, it is a good oil and is also helpful in losing belly fat. In my cooking, I use a little ghee and many dishes I cook without fat, but at the time of eating; I pour a tablespoon of coconut oil in my dish because my body needs fat to function better. People gain weight when they eat packaged food and fried foods very often, and this kind of foods give us weight as well as diseases.

Building Muscle and Losing Body Fat: The contents, which supplements contain, are naturally installed in coconut oil. In supplements those materials are fake and imitation, such as chemicals or steroids, whereas coconut oil possesses the natural ones. It helps burn the fat and good to build up the muscles. One may consume a tablespoon of this oil three times a day and may get real results. You can add to your soup, oatmeal or pour over your cooked food. It enhances the taste of food. You may even eat fresh coconut, but you have to eat a lot, and so far I know; fresh coconut is fattening. But the coconut oil is not fattening.

Perfect for Hair Care: If you want long and thick shiny hair, massage your hair roots with coconut oil when they are wet. In India, women rub their hair with this oil after wash, and they enjoy long thick fat braid, shiny, lustrous hair. It helps remove dandruff, moisture hair, and increase the quantity of your hair. Your hair will look shiny, soft and controlled. Massaging with coconut oil, nourishes the hair follicles, strengthens hair; boosts the health of scalp and the hair, and you will never get pimples or itch in your hair. You may rub a little bit of it between your hands and gently pat your hair to condition and control your hair.

It is Anti-Ageing: Coconut oil helps improve the antioxidant level and can contribute to slow down the aging process as per research published in the Medical journal Food and Function. Coconut oil also promotes reducing stress on our liver and lowers oxidative stress. Coconut oil assists detoxification because of the way it works with the liver. You may take one tablespoon of coconut oil with antioxidant rich blueberries at breakfast and witness the positive results of a naturally slow aging process. My mom applied it directly to her face, neck, hands and arms to moisturize and it softened her skin.

Hormone Balance: Regular consumption of coconut oil benefits your hormones as well. Coconut oil can also promote naturally balance hormones because it is a significant source of saturated fat that carries Lauric Acid. Studies show coconut oil may be an excellent oil to incorporate in our daily food during menopause and also can have potent effects on estrogen level. You may also try to balance hormones naturally by consuming fewer grains and sugar and compensate with healthy fats from coconut flax seeds, avocado, and ghee (You will find 'how to make Ghee' recipe in my other books).

NOTE: - Coconut oil is an amazing oil that does not break down quickly even at the high temperatures like other oils do. It does not go rancid quickly and has excellent nutritional properties and benefits. I never burn it to cook or fry. I always swirl coconut oil on my prepared dishes, such s soups, vegetable dishes, and cooked lintels.

Cucumber

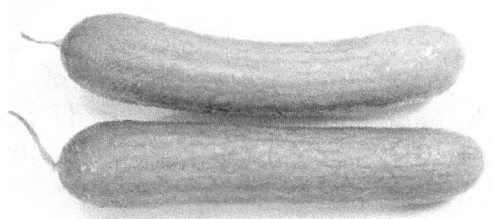

Cucumber is a popular vegetable that belongs to the plant family as pumpkin, squash, celery and watermelon. Cucumber, like watermelon, contains 95 percent of water, which is good for hydration if we frequently consume it in summer. Cucumbers are available all year long, and they contain unique polyphenol and other compounds that can help to reduce the risk of many physical and mental disorders. They are full of nutrients like vitamin K and B vitamins, vitamin C, manganese, potassium, and copper. However, if you regularly consume cucumbers, you may never experience nutrient deficiency.

Helps Fight Inflammation: Cucumbers possess numerous antioxidant properties that may help to soothe the inflammatory condition of the human body. When we have less inflammation in the bones and joints, there are fewer pains and aches in the body, especially knees. Cucumbers also contain the very popular vitamin C and beta-carotene that helps to lower the risk of chronic diseases including heart disease. (Must read an actual story at the end of this chapter).

Freshen Your Breath: Consuming cucumber removes bad mouth odor. In Nature Cure, we believe eating cucumbers may reduce the excess heat in the stomach, which is the primary cause of generating bacteria and produce bad breath in the mouth.

Helps Manage Stress: Cucumbers contain multiple B vitamins, including vitamin B 1, vitamin B 5, and vitamin B 7 (biotin). B vitamins are known to help ease feelings of anxiety and buffer some of the damaging effects of stress.

Protect Your Brain: Cucumbers contain anti-inflammatory properties that appear to play a significant role in brain health. It cleanses the brain and helps keep it calm. Also, we in Nature Cure believe cucumber helps to improve memory and protects nerve cells while we are getting matured.

Helps Kidney Stones: Cucumber juice is full of nutrients. If you consume one cup of cucumber juice three times a day, it helps the kidney stones start dissolving and come out as tiny pieces through the urine tract.

Helps Digestive Health: Cucumbers are highly rich in water and fiber. These are the two most essential elements which the human body craves. If you suffer from acidity, then drinking a lot of water may help to remove the acute symptoms of acidity temporarily, thus giving you less discomfort in the system. There is a possibility that the water-rich cucumbers may assist you in this condition. After trying a couple of days, if you feel it is not working for your system, you can stop consuming them. Also, the skin of cucumbers possess insoluble fiber; that adds roughage to your stool, and that can help a smooth bowel movement.

Helps Lose Weight: We all know cucumbers are very low in calories, yet they are filling and satisfying. Do you know one medium cucumber contains just 16 calories, which is way low. Its soluble fiber dissolves into a gel-like texture in the system to help to slow the digestion. This process helps us to feel full longer, and this is the #1 reason that fiber-rich food helps us to lose weight as well as control weight.

Support Heart Health: Cucumbers contain potassium that contributes to lower blood pressure. A proper balance of potassium both inside and outside the body cells is crucial for your body to function properly. Cucumber, being full of water and fiber is a light food; Thus helping the heart work well.

Make Excellent Healthy Juice: There are several ways to consume cucumbers. You can eat raw in the salads or just cut up into pieces. Cucumber pickle makes a wonderful condiment for your meals. You can make cucumber juice and drink as it is, or add a spoon of honey, lemon juice, or add any other vegetable of your choice. You can also make cucumber juice with fruits or green leaves whatever you prefer, and I tell you that this drink becomes a delicious food and heals the body. It goes into our system and immediately assimilates in the blood channels right away giving us great health and energy. All fruits, vegetables, and green leaves are full of nutrients, minerals, vitamins and enzymes; which make excellent and healthy foods and being all natural, the human body accepts them happily.

NOTE: - Cucumber produces gas and makes **feel bloated to some individuals**. So watch out, if it interrupts your system then try to stay away from it. It also possesses potassium that everyone cannot handle. So please talk to your doctor before you start taking in anything new or in higher quantity.

A true story on Cucumbers:
I have an Aunt in Bangalore, India. She was suffering from acute arthritis. I went from the USA, and I got a chance to meet her after many years. Her fingers and toes were bent and swollen due to an arthritis problem. She was a stunning lady, petite and slim. When I saw her, I walked briskly to hug her, but she stopped me and told me not to touch her as her bones hurt because of extreme pain. She came close to me on my right side and kissed me on my head and blessed my husband and me. After a week, she called me and invited us to lunch. I refused and said, "When I visit India next time we will eat with her family." But she insisted and said she had a maid who did all the cooking, and she wanted me at her place. I had to accept the invitation because she loved us so much.

The maid served the lunch; I was amazed to see she had only a platter full of sliced cucumbers and a variety of food for us on the table. I asked her why she was eating only cucumbers. She explained in detail. Her doctor, a bone specialist, put her on a proper raw diet and told her to choose only one item to eat for three months. I asked her if it was difficult to eat only one vegetable for such a long time and why cucumber? She said that was her favorite vegetable that is why she picked cucumbers and aunt also said that she got used to this new habit. She was motivated to try anything to beat the acute pain.

I visited India again after three years and went to meet that aunt again. I was curious to know about her health. When she saw us, she came running and hugged both of us so hard that tears rolled down on my cheeks due to happiness. The first question I asked was about her arthritis pain. She said "what pain? I am perfectly alright; there's no pain at all".

In Nature Cure, we are taught we can heal and cure our body with the food we eat. Also, we should have that kind of food which is nutritious for our body and does not make our body sick. It is the reason I repeatedly advise my students and friends to consume lots of fresh green leaves, vegetables and fruits because these are full of fiber, vitamins, enzymes, minerals and nutrients. This kind of food cleanses our intestines and helps push out the wastes and toxins that accumulate in our body.

Eggplant

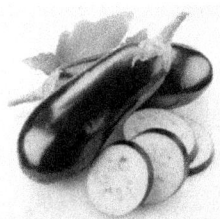

Eggplant is also called aubergine and bringal. Consuming all kinds of fruits and vegetables has proved to reduce the risk of many health disorders. Numerable studies have suggested that increasing consumption of plant foods helps decrease the likelihood of heart disease, obesity, diabetes, heart illness and promotes a great healthy complexion and lustrous hair, increased energy, and lower weight. Because its effects are heat-producing and dryness, try to consume it more in the winter season.

Helps Heart health: Eggplant contains vitamin B-6, vitamin C, the fiber and phytonutrients contents in eggplants and all these compounds support heart health. Regularly eating the foods that contain flavonoid help to lower the risk of heart disorder. Even if you eat small portions of flavonoid-rich foods every day, you may still get benefits and enjoy enhanced health. Numerous studies tell us that anthocyanins content (flavonoid) plays a significant role to lower the risk of health condition and gives energy to the heart.

Help Lower Cholesterol: Researchers, now are saying, the consumption of eggplant may help to lower the bad cholesterol, especially if the patients consume eggplant juice. This juice also may contribute to reducing the weight and blood cholesterol levels.

Helps Heal Hemorrhoids: Eggplant is an excellent vegetable for hemorrhoids. If you are suffering from piles and hang nails, then take the whole top hard part, which connects the eggplant; grind it to a paste and apply to the bottom twice a day daily when you are resting. This process helps reduce the pain and hangnails may dry and fall off the skin in a natural way. Also, try to consume half an eggplant five days a week, cooked as you prefer.

May Help Cancer Patients: The compound anthocyanins in the eggplant vegetable are highly beneficial for cancer patients. This compound, beneficial antioxidants, and anti-inflammatory compounds have the ability to reveal anti-cancer effects. Studies show that all these compounds help protect body cells damaged by free radicals. They also help prevent tumor growth. They stimulate detoxifying enzymes within the cells and contribute to disabling the cancer cells, but one has to consume eggplant with the peel. Anthocyanins are water-soluble pigments that give the eggplant their well-known dark purple complexion.

Helps Reduce Acidity: An anthocyanin within the eggplant skin is a very powerful antioxidant that can help reduce acidity if you are suffering discomfort from bloating, belching and burping. Regularly consuming long sized purple eggplant with the peel; cook the way you like, and eat continuously daily for at least three months. When you are bloated and the feeling of your stomach like a football, will disappear. It can also help you to heal your liver problem.

Weight Management and Satiety: Eggplant contains dietary fiber, which is an important factor to control weight and will also help you experience a feeling of being full for longer time. The compounds in it will contribute to increasing satiety and reduce the appetite, thus consuming a fewer calories; it can help you to satiate your pallet and lower your calorie consumption. Eggplant is low in calories; it can do a great part of a healthy, low-calorie diet. Eggplant skin is full of fiber, potassium and magnesium and antioxidants.

Garlic

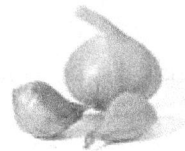

Garlic is an excellent herb, and we all know it very well as a natural health remedy that has long been used to heal various diseases. It is available everywhere and in all seasons. Once you know, its benefits you will like to use it in your daily food. You may consume cooked or fresh. You can easily include it in your food and enjoy a fountain of youth. Do not limit yourself to fresh garlic only. Dry garlic powder or dried garlic flakes are just as efficient and easy to store in the kitchen cabinet for daily use.

As per the recommendations, adults may consume no more than one garlic clove twice a day and the children can eat one-quarter to one-half a clove once or twice a day if needed. Garlic has some amazing abilities to help in our everyday lives. When used for medicinal purposes, Garlic can contribute to healing different kinds of ailments as well as making your dinner amazingly delicious. I, strongly do not recommend to take garlic tablets because while in the manufacturing process, the Allicin compound, the most significant antioxidant and anti-inflammatory content in garlic destroys. If you want to consume raw garlic for an individual reason and do not wish your mouth to smell bad, then soak five or six peeled garlic cloves in water or lassi (yogurt drink) overnight and eat in the morning. This raw garlic will not produce bad breath. It has an endless list of benefits.

Helps Immune System: Winter season is the best time to improve health with the consumptions of garlic; it boosts the immune system and protects you from colds and flu. In the old days, our parents dipped a garlic clove in the honey; chewed and swallowed with hot water or a hot cup of tea. They were hardly sick. We never saw anyone consuming medicines in our family when we were small. I remember, my mom cleaning, grinding and using a lot of garlic while cooking food.

It sounds so funny to say that my mom kept garlic bulbs in the kitchen always and said that was to scare the snakes to enter the house.

Helps Bones: In the case of a broken bone, slipped bone, or long bone, garlic can help to the bone health.

Help Lower Fever: In fever, crush half a bulb of garlic, put in a handkerchief; making a ball and let the patient smell it always. Also, give 5 grams of garlic juice, diluted with double the water to the patient three times a day for a couple of days and this helps lower the high fever.

Helps Stomach Ache: Add one teaspoon of garlic juice in seven teaspoons of lukewarm water and drink it. This garlic juice helps in pushing out the gas and removes stomach ache.

Helps Heart Health: Garlic contains Allicin compound that can kill that dangerous bacteria in the body that even penicillin cannot kill. If one is experiencing a heart attack, give five garlic cloves to the patient and let him chew and swallow. The waiting for the help will be worth as the effects of garlic will delay the attack. The accumulated gas passes out after one eats garlic and you can give garlic boiled in the milk also if the help is not yet there. Regularly consuming garlic improves heart health and makes it healthy. It helps remove plaque deposits that gathers on the walls of human body's veins. The consumption of garlic can bring incredible benefits for heart disorder.

Helps Arthritis: Being rich in anti-oxidants, anti-inflammatory contents, and Vitamin C, garlic helps decrease inflammation in the joints and body, thus helping arthritis patients to sooth and get relief from pain. Besides eating garlic, you can also cook half a crushed garlic bulb in half a cup of sesame seed oil until garlic completely burns. Cool it down and strain. You can massage your aching areas with this garlic oil and get some relief. If your ear hurts, even then you can pour 4 or 5 drops of this garlic oil in your ear twice a day and get relief.

Help Babies Gain Weight: When you are pregnant, and the baby is weak, consuming one garlic clove twice a day, will help you to have a healthy baby.

Hyperthyroid Conditions: Garlic possesses a high level of iodine that helps in healing hyperthyroid conditions. Herbalists swear by this herb and treat their patients with garlic for several mental and physical conditions.

Help Lower Blood Pressure: If one consumes seven drops of garlic juice mixed with seven drops of water twice a day for a longer period; it contributes to lower the high blood pressure and energize your body. When I was in the Nature Cure School in India, I noticed my therapy instructor had some fresh little garlic cloves on her table always. So I asked her the reason; she said that she had high blood pressure and did not want to eat any medicine. She munched on those garlic cloves off and on.

Helps Scurvy Disease: Garlic contains a high level of Vitamin C, and this vitamin can heal the scurvy condition in the body. Adults mostly get this problem in matured age due to the lake of consumption of fruits and vegetables. Children, sometimes, also get the scurvy condition due to avoiding eat greens. Since garlic is full of Vitamin C, individuals suffering from this disease can take help of garlic any time they desire.

Help Cancer Patients: Garlic possesses Vitamin B6, which is said to have cancer-fighting abilities. Check with your doctor for advice because herbalists give garlic to their cancer patients. They believe Garlic is a potent herb, and it can assist to prevent multiple types of cancers, like stomach cancer, breast cancer, colon cancer, bladder cancer and prostate cancer. Herbalists also believe that garlic is capable of reducing the tumors if treated with it.

Helps Diabetics: Garlic is highly equipped with anti-oxidants and a content Allicin that help regulates the blood sugar as it enhances the insulin level in the blood. Diabetic patients, who regularly consume garlic, get to control their blood sugar.

Helps Maintain Youthfulness: Garlic, being an extremely nutrient herb increases your hunger. It is good for those, who have lost their appetite. Regular Consumption of raw garlic clove with honey twice a day, helps increase body strength, boosts sex life, heals disorders, and you feel youthful. It also improves your digestive power, you maintain youthfulness and show few wrinkles even when you got matured. Regular consumption of garlic increases longevity and pushes away the old age.

NOTE: - For any reason if you consume raw garlic, then either take in juice or diluted with water or take a pea size garlic paste and swallow with water. If you consume raw crushed, paste, or juice alone, then **it will burn your windpipe, and you will feel the burn as it travels inside you. It gives you a highly discomfort and unbearable feeling. Also, do not take a large dose, it can prove detrimental to your body and your health. It may also produce a disagreeable odor.** After enjoying a meal with garlic, chew on some fresh cilantro leaves or coriander seeds to eliminate the lovely aroma of garlic breath.

If you need more information about garlic, then you read a book written by Yoshio Koto "Garlic, The Unknown Miracle Worker."

Ginger Root

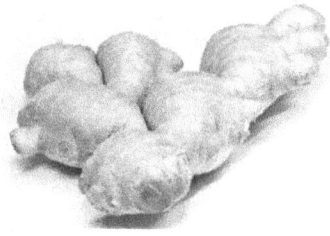

Researchers now have confirmed ginger root helps to reduce the nausea conditions such as morning sickness, postoperative disturbance, and chemotherapy treatments. Nature has provided many vegetables and fruits for the benefits of people and some of them have exceedingly good qualities built in them to cure certain diseases. Ginger is one the roots which is highly beneficial for every human being. Arabians, Asians and Chinese have been using this herb from ancient times for food as well as medicines. Ginger is used in many forms such as ground, dried powder and Julian to flavor curry dishes, soups, pickles, sauces, chutneys, bread, confections, and tea.

Soothes Inflammation: Ginger is highly equipped with anti-inflammatory properties which contributes to reducing pain and inflammation, in managing arthritis, migraines and headaches, backache and menstrual cramps. Add half a spoon of ghee in one spoon of ginger juice and consume it with a half cup of lukewarm water twice a day. Take one dose early morning; the second dose at bedtime for at least three weeks and do not take anything before and after for 30 minutes. Ginger may also help prevent stomach ulcers caused by anti-inflammatory drugs, such as aspirin and ibuprofen.

Heart Health: Research by the Ayurvedic pundits shows the gingerroot has enough qualities like it gives warmth to a human body as well its antioxidants stimulates the blood circulation. It is full of nutrients and bioactive compounds that have powerful benefits for your health, body and brain. If your heart is weak, you feel lazy and small; by taking half a cup of ginger fusion with a pinch of salt every day; will help you feel energetic and healthy. To make a ginger fusion, boil one teaspoonful of ginger powder in a cup of water and let it cook until half the water burns. It is suitable for winter but in the summer season take only in the morning.

Helps Fight Allergies - Flu and Common Cold: Ginger is dry and warm by nature and is used a lot in the winter season. It helps keep the body warm and protects in, sore throat, flu, and common colds. Ginger tea is very popular in the Indian community. Whether someone is sick or not in the house, we still keep on drinking ginger tea to protect ourselves from cold waves. We use in every dish for its flavor and benefits.

Helps In Loose Motion: If you are suffering from diarrhea, take half a cup of boiling water; add one spoon of ginger juice and drink every hour until diarrhea stops. Its main job is to push out toxins of the body, clear the intestinal tract; it helps reduce gas and painful spasms.

Soothes Cough: For severe coughing take equal ratio amounts of ginger juice and honey four times a day for relief. Mix rock sugar powder 100 grams, ginger powder 100 grams, mulathi powder 100 grams, black pepper powder 50 grams and one spoon of honey. Take half a spoon of this mixture with lukewarm water four times a day. Try to stay indoors to protect your chest and neck from the cold. This herbal medicine is very effective; continue taking this mixture for at least seven days. You can make more if needed.

Helps Flatulence and Colic: I use ginger as a vegetable, herb and as well as medicine. It dramatically helps heal flatulence and colic. One drop of ginger juice mixed with one tablespoon of water and a little honey, if given to small babies when they cry with a colic (gas) problem: it helps sooth their pain. Also, it is better than pharmaceutical medicine and no additional side effects. Adults, who suffer from indigestion, store excessive gas in the digestive tract that may be the result of undigested foods, lactose intolerance, or the consumption of certain foods that are not compatible with their systems. They become the victims of flatulence. Their system produces waste gas during digestion, and they mostly keep on releasing gas. It is a common problem in obesity. The regular consumption of ginger in any form you prefer will help.

During pregnancy: You can put ginger pieces in salted and diluted vinegar and suck on it anytime of the day when you desire. Try it in your hot soups and tea using a little honey that will energize you. You can also nibble crystallized ginger if you are nauseated or feel like throwing. It will help pass the gas and push out toxins giving you a feeling of relief.

The ginger root grows under the soil like potatoes and carrots. Its smell is aromatic and penetrating. Its taste is biting and spicy hot. It was cultivated originally in India and China. Records say ginger came from Spain and was established as a commercial crop in Jamaica only two thousand years ago. We all know its medicinal properties and in Nature Cure, ginger is beneficial for many patients suffering from many diseases like asthma, cancer, colitis, weight loss, and diabetes. One tablespoon of ginger juice and one teaspoon of honey mixed and swallowed ¾ times a day may be very helpful in disorders as mentioned above. Its primary job is to push out the toxins of the human body and cleanse the digestive system. BUT REMEMBER, IN SUMMER, ONE SHOULD TAKE A SMALL AND MILD DOSE OF GINGER AS ITS EFFECTS ARE DRY AND HOT.

Goji Berries

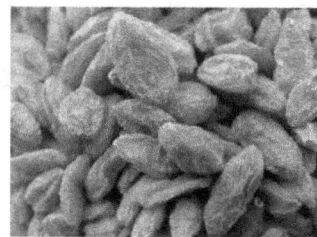

Goji berries contain vitamin C, vitamin A, high antioxidant compounds and are the super food. Some people also call it wolfberries. It looks like cherry tomatoes and the size of the tip of your little finger. It has a bright orange-red color that comes from the shrubs of the Himalayas and China. In India, people have been eating goji berries for generations believing it increases longevity. In China and India, the herbalists give goji berries to their patients to eat fresh, brew in tea, make liquid extracts, and add to their soups. In Nature Cure, we believe these berries are highly nutrient, regular consumption of this fruit keeps us healthy and young. Herbalists use goji berries to treat many different health problems. Now they are available as dried, goji berry trail mix, juice, and tea and you may add to your oatmeal, cream of wheat, and salads. These are an expensive product but equipped with high nutrients and antioxidants compound. I have heard goji berry supplements are also available, but I have not seen yet.

Help Sleep Being rich in nutrients, people believe Goji berries possess calming effects. One feels relaxed and experiences a feeling of being healthy and active. They can perform better with their day to day challenges and sleep well.

High Blood Pressure: Because of the rich nutrients and antioxidants properties that appear in these berries, it promotes to help stabilize the blood pressure level, but you can eat only ten pieces a day. Also, you have to check with your doctor so that it does not interfere with the current medication you are consuming.

Lose Weight: People in Nature Cure believe if you stay healthy and vibrant, you do not gain weight. In simple words if you eat berries and live a healthy life, then there is nothing to worry about weight and cholesterol. I believe goji berries boost our health and promote weight-loss.

Help Vision: When I was in India in 2011, my folks suggested for me to buy some dried goji berries for my family, and I got a list of great benefits. They told me that these are excellent for the health of our eyes, especially for older generations, and I brought some with me. It also promotes sharpening eyesight. I mixed them in the yogurt and left in the kitchen for a couple of hours. By the time it was ready, the berries were soft, and my husband and I enjoyed our breakfast.

Diabetes: These berries are sweet and little tangy like raisins, but its sweetness is 100% natural, so it does not increase your blood sugar level if consumed in moderation. You can talk to your doctor before you start taking anything new for the safety of your health. If you eat 10 to 13 goji berries every day, they support to strengthen your immune system, cleanse the liver and you enjoy better health.

Alzheimer's: Goji berries possess vitamin C, vitamin A, and antioxidant compounds, which help purify the blood and give energy to the patient. We also believe it boosts memory. These berries are best as an aid in the treatment or use them as a prevention to stay healthy. Its juice and smoothie are delicious and very live foods. It helps decrease fatigue and boost energy.

Immune system: A small research published in the Journal of Medicinal Food In 2009, showed goji berries can improve the function of metabolism, strengthen the immune system, improve circulation and lift the mood.

Slow Off Aging And Fatigue: Our body cells die and generate new cells as a natural process to repair the body. While maturing, the body cells drop the energy, start limping; cling to each other, become clusters and lifeless. If one eats goji berries regularly, it helps the cells to start loosening up, get separated, and come to a natural form. Thus giving vitality and energy to the dying cells and make them healthy. So, if we consume a few goji berries every day as medicine, it can do a fantastic job. In my family, it is "A fountain of youth." When I was buying these berries in India, the store owner advised me to eat 15 pieces daily to stay healthy and energized.

NOTE: - Goji berries grew in abundance on the evergreen shrubs in the Himalaya's valleys, and hills in the remote areas of India and pesticides were not used. This berry can interrupt and harm you if you are taking blood thinner, blood pressure, or cholesterol medicine. Consult your doctor before starting to take anything new.

Grapes

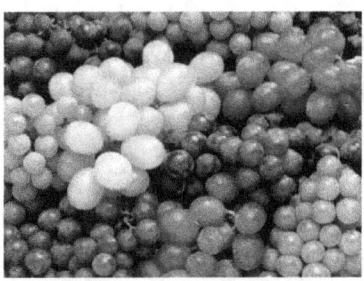

Grapes are the most popular and delicious fruits on this earth. They are highly rich in vitamins A, C, B6, and foliate. Also, grapes contain essential minerals like calcium, iron, phosphorus, selenium and magnesium. Grapes possess very potent antioxidants well-known flavonoids, which can help decrease the damage done by free radicals and slow aging process. Grapes play a significant role in promoting a healthy and youthful life. Regular consumption of fruits and vegetables of all kinds is a sure short way to reduce the risk of diabetes, heart disease, diabetes, cancer and indigestion and many other physical conditions.

Asthma: Regular consumption of grapes helps asthma patients to strengthen the lungs and soothe a cough. The high content of anti-oxidants that appears in the skins of red grapes is highly beneficial for lung patients. If you juice red grapes, then do not throw the peels (roughage), because the surface is mostly wet with juice and has nutrients and fiber, that is what human body needs. You may grind them and use any way you can. The kind of polyphenol contents grapes contains is very beneficial for asthma patients. If someone gets blood spots in the spit, even then grapes help to stable the condition and asthma patient eventually feels better.

Help Inflammation: The dynamic contents in grapes, work as an anti-inflammatory agent that may help to turn down the inflammation, and it may be useful for heart disease and reduce pains and aches in the joints. Grapes have the capability to push out the toxins from the body.

Help Easy Teething: When your small baby is going through a difficult time during teething, give them one tablespoon of fresh grape juice four times a day for easy teething and the baby will cry less.

Heart Disease: Grapes are the rich sources of flavonoids, the natural anti-inflammatory contents that have shown the right results of reducing the risk of bad cholesterol (LDL). The high content of polyphenol in grapes may help decrease the possibility of heart disease by preventing plaque build-up and reduce the blood pressure also. I believe consuming grapes on a regular basis strengthens the heart and helps not to have plaque accumulation in the arteries. If someone is suffering from nervousness or weakness of heart condition, eating 15 to 20 grapes every day like medicine, or drinking 6 oz. of fresh grape juice twice a day, may help the patient feel healthy and stable. Juice is better as it assimilates in the blood channels immediately. In Nature Cure, we believe it is better to eat healthy food as prevention and consume fewer medicines later.

As per the studies, grapes contain fiber and potassium that support heart health. I further believe an increase in potassium intake along with a decrease in sodium consumption is the most important change a person can make an effort to reduce the risk of heart disease.

Help Reduce weight: Studies have shown that regularly consuming plant foods like grapes decrease the risk of being obese and most people live a longer life. Grapes also include powerful components that make them even more essential and valuable for human health. We call grapes "super food" because they reduce the risk of many health conditions. Consuming 15 grapes five minutes before each meal is the first step towards losing weight however you have to eat daily to see results.

Help Cancer: Grapes contain quercetin that is a powerful anti-oxidant that may help show the anti-cancer effects, but more studies are being done consistently so that more positive results can be confirmed. Grapes contain polyphenol compound; that is a powerful anti-oxidant agent that may help to slow down different kinds of cancer, such as lung, colon, mouth, pancreatic, and prostate cancer.

High Blood Pressure: Grapes are a very nutritious food and come in a variety of colors. They are equally rich in potassium and antioxidant. Especially, people with high blood pressure can be benefited by the consumption of grapes.

Helps Constipation: Regularly eating foods rich in water content like grapes, cucumbers, watermelon and cantaloupe help you hydrate and promote smooth bowel movements. Grapes also possess high fiber, especially the black ones, which is important to eliminate constipation.

Helps Cough: Eating grapes boost energy to the lungs. It helps heal a cough and reduce the mucus. Try to consume only sweeter grapes during a cough, and drink no water after eating them. Grapes are given to patients suffering from any lung disease because grapes boost health and energy.

Help Soothe Allergies: Grapes also contribute to decreasing symptoms of allergies like watery eyes, running nose and frequent colds. In Nature Cure, if someone is suffering from cold, we suggest the patient consume approximately 25 grapes twice a day. Grapes help soothe the sneezing and the sinus too.

Helps Increase Milk For Nursing Mothers: If a nursing mother cannot produce more milk and the baby stays hungry, then the mother may eat grapes every day. She will start to produce more milk to satisfy the baby.

Alzheimer's disease: Grapes are highly equipped with antioxidants that appear to be helpful for healing Alzheimer's disease. In Natural Treatment, grapes are recommended to women with hot flashes and mood swing conditions. It also helps stable blood glucose. It is the world's healthiest food on earth.

Honey

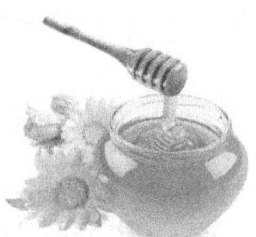

I like honey's second name, "liquid gold." It is an excellent food with an unending list of valuable benefits of nutrients. I migrated to the US in 1978, and after almost ten years; suffering so much from a car accident I went back home to India to learn Yoga, Breathing Exercises, Meditation, and Nature Cure. The first advice my teacher gave me was to bring honey in my life. I told him I have four kinds of honey into my life; my wonderful husband and my three lovely daughters and he said I needed the fifth one to make my life sweeter. When I came back to the USA, I started consuming a little bit of it which I later realize it is a powerhouse of benefits.

We, in Nature Cure, call honey "Yogavahi," which means it enhances and strengthens all other herbs and processes in the body. It also has the quality of penetrating the deepest tissues of the body and naturally helps physical and mental problems. It is considered a vehicle which enhances the potency of the different kinds of medicines when combined with it. And people believe it is great for the health of their body, mind, and longevity. Though Natural Treatments show results slowly, they do work and are 100% natural. When we use honey with other herbal preparations, it enhances the medicinal qualities of those preparations and contributes to reaching the deeper tissues of the body. It is one of the world's power foods which should be in every kitchen. I would love to share some of its benefits. It is the only food produced by insects and consumed by human beings. It comes readymade and needs no cooking. It is also sweeter than table sugar and can last for literally centuries if stored properly.

Lose Weight: Sugar has empty calories that promote health issues and obesity, but honey is having significant benefits contributes to reducing the fatty build up in the cardiovascular system. Also, refined sugar or sucrose ferments in our stomach to cause any harm from bacterial invasion, whereas honey does not ferment and, therefore, does not generate any disorder. It contains natural nutrients and antioxidants that are believed to be an ideal fuel for burning body fat while we sleep.

Alzheimer's disease: Honey possesses a unique antioxidant known as 'pinocembrin,' which is not present in other products. This novel compound is believed to aid in curing Alzheimer's disease. It also helps to reduce oxidative stress. Scientists are also looking forward to helping heal patients with dementia, stroke, and Alzheimer's disease successfully.

Works as a Probiotic: Honey, has been said, is full of good bacteria, but some varieties of honey have significant amounts of friendly bacteria. The human body needs this good bacteria. When you take a teaspoon of honey first thing in the morning and do not eat or drink anything for 30 minutes, it boosts and increases energy and gives you the strength to fight infections, if you get any. It has therapeutic properties.

Skin Glow: Its anti-bacterial qualities are very useful for the skin and when you add other ingredients, such as yogurt, lemon, turmeric, olive oil, grape seed oil, or oat bran; can exfoliate, moisturize and nourish your skin and bring a glow to it! For home beauty treatment, you do not have to go out; simply look in your kitchen and you will find everything.

Cancer: Honey possesses flavonoids, antioxidants, and unique benefits that contribute to decreasing the risk of some cancers. Cancer patients are given honey in small quantities.

Possesses Iron: Its valuable properties of iron, sodium, manganese, silica, calcium, potassium, phosphorus, sulfur, iodine, carotene and antibiotic compounds give a boost to human health. It is like a tonic and medicine. Not too many people know its benefits. Taking a spoon of honey first thing in the morning in warm water can keep you energetic and enhance your health. Herbalists have been using it as a medium in combination with other medicines. Be sure it is the real one!

Ulcers and Other G.I. Disorders: Honey can be an excellent treatment and may assist the ulcers and bacterial gastroenteritis. It is the one sweetener which is not man-made or processed and contains antibacterial qualities and treats humans effectively.

It is Anti-bacterial and Anti-fungal: All the honey available is antibacterial because the bees include an enzyme during the process of its production. It contains potassium that helps kill the bacteria which generates diseases, such as bronchitis pneumonia and Typhoid. If someone is suffering from this type of illness, then regular consumption of honey, helps faster healing.

Increases athletic performance: In olden times, athletes ate honey, dates, and dried figs to improve their performance. In the small towns and villages of India, athletes still use honey as they know how and from where to collect it. It is better and superior in maintaining glycogen levels and improves recovery time than the other sweeteners available on the market. Athletes prefer honey as a sweetener over the other products on the market because it is a concentrated source of fructose and glucose which enhances our health.

Regulates Blood Sugar: Though Honey contains simple sugars, yet we believe it is not the same as regular white sugar, substitutes, or artificial sweeteners. It is an exact combination of glucose and fructose that helps the body regulate blood sugar level. There are different varieties of honey, and some of them have a low hypoglycemic index, and they do not shake your blood sugar. We also consider it a light food.

Coughs and Throat Irritations: Honey contributes to the soothing of the coughs, especially if used with basil, ginger powder and the juice of a lemon. Children get great results faster when they take a couple of doses of it for the relief of a cough or throat irritation. Nature Cure therapists suggest honey to children for minor colds, coughs, and allergies than over the counter medicines. Mix 1 oz.

glycerin in a glass jar with 3 oz. honey and the juice of one boiled lemon. Mix it and store in a glass bottle. Take one teaspoon four times a day and you may get relief from a cough in three days.

Promotes Sleep: Because of its sedative effects, even a cup of warm water with a spoon of honey promotes sleep and soothes the throat. You may take a tablespoon of honey in a cup of not too hot water with the juice of a lemon and enjoy a good night sleep. In a cup of warm milk, a spoon of honey also promotes sleep, but this is for those individuals who want to put on some weight.

Heals wounds and burns: It is also useful for external use. Some people use honey on irritated or bruised skin. External application of it has shown to be effective as a regular use on the affected skin. Make a thin paste of honey and wheat flour; spread on a piece of clean cloth with a butter knife and place over the irritated or affected skin. Next morning wet it with a little warm water and remove. You will see the result in three days. In Nature Cure, we consider it to be the most superior treatment for burns and wounds as it relieves us from pain efficiently and contributes to healing faster with fewer scars.

NOTE: - Doctor D. C. Jarvis is the author of a book 'Folk Medicine' in which you can find more detail about using honey to enhance the healing power.

In India, Ayurvedic practitioners have been using honey in their medicines for centuries, and they believed in its benefits which contributed in healing various ailments. It is also said to be useful in improving eyesight, nausea, weight loss, curing impotence, urinary tract disorders, bronchial asthma, diarrhea, and body balancing.

Kale

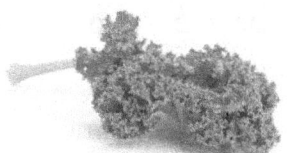

Kale, 'the powerhouse of nutrients' and 'the queen of greens' is the most famous herb at these modern times. It has the highest level of fiber, Vitamin A, Vitamin C, antioxidants, omega-3 acids and high calcium. Kale has no calorie; it is high in fiber and includes no fat. It is great to contribute to digestion and elimination with the high fiber contents it possesses. You may juice it, make a smoothie, sauté it; the choice is yours. My daughter Seema sautés green cabbage. Two minutes before it is tender, she adds a handful chopped kale, and when done she adds one egg. What a great way to enjoy healthy breakfast!

Heart Health: Because of its high antioxidants, consuming kale on a daily basis helps lower the cholesterol level. It also helps in restricting the build-up plaque in the arteries, but you must consult your doctor for advice before eating kale. Studies are underway for exceptional results, but herbalists, in India, use kale for patients, who suffer from indigestion, lung diseases, and mouth cavity cancers.

Vision health: Vitamin A is an excellent support agent for your vision and your skin. It helps enhance the eyesight and eyes health.

Lose Weight: Kale is high in fiber and low in calorie, and includes zero fat. It is filling and satisfying. If you consume a cup of kale in any way, it has only 36 calories, high fiber and no fat at all. It stimulates the metabolism and assists in the elimination of its high fiber content. It maintains regularity and is full of so many nutrients, vitamins, minerals, enzymes, foliate, and magnesium. It aids to lose weight if regularly consumed.

Help Cancers: We all know kale is full of potent antioxidants. The antioxidants, like flavonoids, assist in protecting against many different types of cancers. We all should eat kale as prevention. I use a couple of kale leaves in my juice or a smoothie. I also mix a few leaves of kale thinly sliced in my wheat, barley, corn and millet flours; knead them together with green pepper and sliced onions and make dough with warm water. My paratha (Indian Tortilla) comes out delicious.

Anti-inflammatory Benefits: Kale is very famous for its high anti-inflammatory benefits. If you consume one full cup of kale, it carries a lot of the omega-3 fatty acids; that promotes the fight against asthma, arthritis, and autoimmune disorders.

High in Vitamin C: Kale is very helpful for your immune system, your metabolism, and your hydration.

High in calcium: If you compare kale with milk, then kale has more calcium than milk that assists in preventing bone loss, preventing osteoporosis damage and maintains a healthy metabolism. Vitamin C also promotes to maintain cartilage and joint problems.

Great detoxifying: Kale includes a lot of fiber and sulfur; both are excellent contents to detoxify the body and aid the liver to stay healthy.

High in iron: Kale has an essential and highly requirement of iron for the human body, that helps proper functioning of the body. It supports the formation of hemoglobin, enzymes, and taking oxygen to different body parts. It also helps in cell growth, proper liver function and much more. It is also helpful for the anemic ladies.

High in Vitamin K: Kale is also highly loaded with vitamin K and consuming a diet high in Vitamin K can contribute to protecting against many types of different cancers. It is also essential for a variety of physical functions like normal bone health and blood clotting. Kale with high fiber and increased level of Vitamin K can support individuals suffering from Alzheimer's disease.

NOTE: - As mentioned above, kale contains a high level of Vitamin K, and it works wonders for aiding heals many diseases. Before start consuming kale, please consult your doctor for sincere advice, because Vitamin K can also interrupt your system if you are consuming medicines for certain conditions such as heart disorder (Warfarin), high blood pressure, diabetes, and indigestion. Also, if you consume more kale than you need, it can generate a thyroid problem. Individuals, who have a thyroid condition, stay away from kale.

Kokum (Mangosteen)

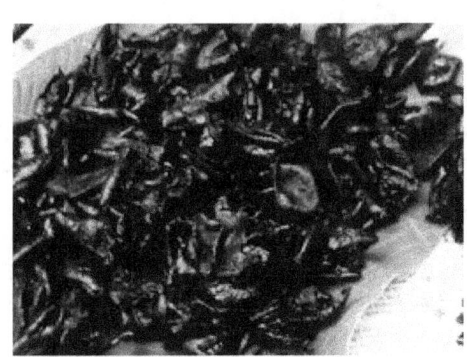

Kokum (mangosteen) is an excellent fruit like a plum, but too sour. Fresh product is never available, so you will find dried kokum, which comes in packets and it is too salty. Dried Kokum looks like dried prunes and plums. It grows in abundance in India; the farmers harvest it twice a year, and it is available everywhere in India because Indian women use it a lot in their cooking. The Kokum farming requires a special care and appropriate handling. This superb fruit is full of medicinal properties. With the help of kokum, herbalists are treating several patients, who are suffering from mental and physical disorders. We all are familiar, how much people like and appreciate the mangosteen (Kokum) juice for its medicinal properties in the whole world!

I cook food at home and feed my family. I do not drink prepackaged juice. I purchase Kokum (mangosteen) from the Indian or the Asian stores. I soak it in water overnight; make a paste next day adding a little water and store it in the refrigerator. Once kokum paste is ready, I make my juice for an exceptional taste with little honey, little mint paste, little ginger juice and artificial sweetener and utilize it in different ways I need.

Consuming half a teaspoon of this paste before breakfast or before going to bed is very helpful to take care of many physical problems. Kokum mixed with cilantro paste and amlika powder helps cure hemorrhoids. It helps fight infection, lose weight, depression, lower cholesterol, digestion, hypertension, urinary track and improve prostate health. If regularly consumed, it aids in improving skin health; induces better sleep, given to cancer patients, to boost the immune system, prevent kidney stones and stay young.

We all know how much mangosteen juice is famous, but it is very expensive. I use Kokum as its natural form, pure and concentrate and it is very inexpensive. I do not believe in purchasing expensive prepackaged stuff and invite unexpected mental or physical disorders.

Immune System: Studies declare it a super fruit due to its unending healing properties and it can assist in strengthening the immune system, healthy metabolism, and indigestion. Herbalists use kokum for treating their patients for fighting infection, depression and digestion and call it an immune system booster.

Heart Health: A small dose of kokum, like half a cup of kokum homemade juice, if consumed every morning, and then one can experience calm and relaxed because of its potent anti-oxidant properties. It also helps lower cholesterol, strengthens the immune system and supports heart health.

Lose Weight: I, once, consumed kokum homemade juice for three months to experience its effects, and I discovered, it promotes to suppress hunger, lowers cholesterol and lose weight. I felt more energized, mentally and physically elevated and lost four pounds. It also helps remove constipation.

Disables Cancer Cells: Kokum which is very high in anti-bacterial plant compound and anti-cancer kokum, assists to block the cancer cell's ability to reach the healthy cell to aid stop cancer bacteria for spreading. Because of its potent anti-inflammatory compound and antioxidants, it contributes as the anti-tumor agent.

Alzheimer's Disease: Studies have found kokum fruit is energy and immune system booster and very helpful in preventing many diseases like diabetes, heart disease, Alzheimer's disease, and other chronic diseases.

Diabetes: Kokum is a powerhouse with a high level of anti-oxidants, can aid support health of diabetic patients and stabilizes the sugar level. Individuals, who are health conscious, can consume kokum (mangosteen) as preventative support.

Nutritional Yeast

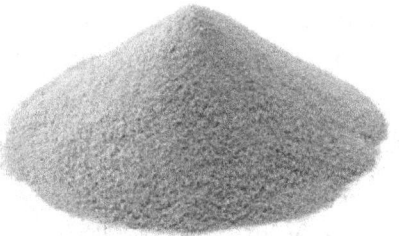

My sister-in-law, Roma, lives in India and her cousin Praveen is a knowledgeable Major in the military, resides in Lucknow, India. He introduced me to consuming yeast. I met Praveen in December 1997 when my husband and I were on a trip to New Delhi, India. He was also vacationing. I noticed Praveen talked a lot about the benefits of yeast and natural health, and I was little skeptical about yeast at that time. When Roma told me that her Aunt was very sick and, doctors felt she could survive for few months. There was panic in the house. This lady was a dance teacher. All her life she was active, but some disease pulled her down, and she ended up in the bed. She called her son Praveen and told him to come and meet her as there was not much time left. He said, "I will only come if you will listen to me." She agreed.

When he reached home, he told his mom she would not eat food for three days, and these were her fasting days. This lady wanted to be with her son all the time as she presumed her death was close. He put her on nutritional yeast, two tablespoons three times a day. He gave her each dose with a tall glass of water, morning, noon and night and she drank a lot of water the whole day. After three days Praveen gave his mom 2 oz. of fresh orange juice three times a day with the regular dose of yeast. The second day she had 4 oz. of orange juice three times a day, and the third day 6 oz. of orange juice three times a day. After six days she told Praveen, she felt better health-wise, but her body was weak. She ate Mung bean daal and one tortilla (roti) made with mixed grains as her main meal for two days and then she started her regular meals. She was in perfect health, regained her energy and began her dancing career again and lived for years. It is the power of Nutritional Yeast!

Detoxify The Body: It is an excellent cleansing agent. One can try to consume for one month and see the results. You feel cleansed internally and at the same time, your Vitamin B intake increases that enhances the level of your energy and health.

Nutritional Yeast is-all-cure agent that can help healing any mental and physical diseases. It is used in cooking, baking, and in the medicines. It is useful for the patients with diabetes, flu, skin eruptions, diarrhea, acne, common cold and lung problems such as respiratory tract infections and much more. Companies also have also been used as a source of Vitamin B, protein and chromium.

Lose Weight: Being rich in fiber, it stimulates the digestive system, strengthens metabolism, and maintains regularity. When you are pushing out your toxins of the body on a daily basis, you lose some pounds and do not gain weight at all.

Diabetic Patients: Because of its chromium content, it helps lower blood glucose with diabetes and chromium also contributes to the body to use insulin more efficiently and bring blood sugar level down. If you regularly consume yeast, it helps push out the toxins from your body and prevent for intense sugar cravings and blood sugar swings.

Constipation: Nutrition yeast promotes to flush out the waste and toxins of the body quickly. It softens the stool and make a natural bowel movement. It stimulates the digestive system, and you do not feel sluggish anymore.

Diarrhea: Nutritional yeast stimulates intestinal enzymes that promote to relieve from diarrhea.

It Is Anti-Aging: Being rich in Vitamin B, Fiber, low-glycemic food, anti-inflammatory proteins pushes out toxins, and numerous minerals make this yeast anti-aging agent. When it can keep us healthy, we do not invite mental and physical disorders, and we stay young, healthy and vibrant. Ayurvedic practitioners call it anti-aging agent.

Common Cold: It promotes to fight bacteria that generate infections in the intestine, as well as it safeguards the body against viral lung infections such as common colds and flu.

Boost Health: Being rich in Vitamin B and protein, nutritional yeast is beneficial for using in cooking the food. It is an incredibly health-promoting agent for vegetarians like us, who live on a plant-based diet.

Eating enough fresh food, low-glycemic foods, regular meals, getting adequate anti-inflammatory proteins in the diet, and consuming a little fat throughout the day are all crucial for taking care of your blood sugar. These are the main principles that will help prevent those blood sugar swings, intense sugar cravings, and prevent symptoms related to blood sugar imbalances such as moodiness, anxiety, fatigue, and headaches. However, you also need to focus on specific nutrients to take care of your blood sugar too.

Low Glycemic: It is a low glycemic food. It contains no added sugar and has low carbohydrates. When we eat unhealthy food, indulge in overeating, or skipping meals; lead to spike the blood levels high and low rapidly, but consuming low glycemic foods such as nutritional yeast, fiber-rich food, whole food, and plant-based foods is essential to manage blood sugar and for healthy living.

Right Nutrients for the Body: The nutrients, most needed by the body for a healthy metabolism are found abundantly in plant-based foods and nutritional yeast that contain the right nutrients. It requires two tablespoons of yeast to swallow with water twice a day, and if you are sick, then you may increase a dose.

Rich In Protein: Nutritional yeast is highly rich in Vitamin B that is an excellent source of amino acids with a complete protein source. It includes the essential amino acids that the human body is not able to produce on its own, but along with all these amino acids, this body can produce on its own. Two tablespoons of Nutritional Yeast possess 8 grams of protein, which you can found in half a cup of lentils or beans. It carries the lowest calories of protein as compared to all other proteins out there and do not be amazed if I tell you, two tablespoons of it contains only 45 calories. Protein and amino acids are the rich sources for body and muscle building blocks in life.

High Fiber: Fiber is another beneficial compound which promotes to slow down the absorption of natural sugars from our food into the bloodstream. Two tablespoons of this yeast carry four grams of fiber. It cleanses the unsafe fats and cholesterol, along with toxins in our body that keep our hearts healthy. The human body needs 25-35 grams of fiber a day; we can add up our daily quota with Nutritional yeast and consume other foods like broccoli, kale, avocado, apples and pears, oats, barley, whole grains and beans. Food, rich in fiber gives us a feeling of fullness, stimulates the digestive system; maintains regularity and makes us healthy. The best thing is we never gain weight.

Rich in Minerals: Nutritional yeast is a rich source of numerous minerals and includes zinc and magnesium. Both the minerals are essential for the blood sugar. Herbalists believe it as a powerhouse nutrient and is crucial to maintaining good heart, metabolic, mental, bone, and digestive health. Some other best sources include lentils and beans, whole grains, greens, legumes, and some other foods like almonds, cashews, along with coconut and its products, avocados, and some fruits and vegetables. Nutritional yeast contains magnesium which is good for a small serving, but zinc is the real mineral star found in nutritional yeast. It is incredibly important for your blood sugar, your overall energy, immune health, and weight. Nutritional yeast includes in just two tablespoons.

Vitamin B: Nutritional yeast is high in Vitamin B. Vitamin B helps the human body to use carbohydrates for energy. It also promotes to prevent blood sugar swings. Two tablespoons of this yeast possess 9.5 milligrams of Thiamin, 9. milligrams of Riboflavin, 56 milligrams of Niacin, 9.6 milligrams of Vitamin B6, 240 micrograms of Folate, and 7.7 micrograms of Vitamin B12. Remember all different kinds of yeasts are rich sources of natural Vitamin B, because they grow on B-rich bacteria in the soil (such as Vitamin B12). But do not try to get your Vitamin B 12 from yeast alone. Here is a smart choice to eat as many other vitamin B products as you can and do not get a habit to the ready-made supplements to make you healthy.

For vegetarians, it is essential to eat those kinds of foods which contain all the B Vitamins; incorporate into your daily meals and live healthy with no disease.

In Nature Cure, we believe we require these foods to optimal brain and memory function that prevents depression and mania and iron intake, and manganese is crucial for all aspects of our health.

Yeast contributes to convert food into energy, reduce blood sugar, make and break down those fatty acids,that we need for our healthy hair, skin, and nails. As said before, it also emerges with Vitamin B-12 and Vitamin C to utilize proteins; is essential for healthy brain and memory development, and for healthy red blood cell formation. It is important for pregnant women as they need enough of energy and strength.

Papaya

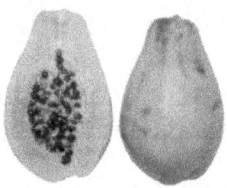

Papaya is a fruit and available throughout the year. It has a rich, delicious sweet taste with a soft consistency of butter. When I was in school and lived with my parents in India, there were two papaya trees which produced lots of high-quality fruits. My mom used to send my brother to deliver those papayas to my relative's and friend's houses. Each piece was huge; maybe around 5 - 8 lbs. Each piece contained a few seeds, and its flesh was sweet and delicious. I have eaten the best papaya in my life, and in large quantities. The inside flesh is a rich orange in color with a slight yellow shade. Papaya is full of great benefits for skin, health, and hair. Not just the fruit itself, but other parts of papaya also are very beneficial. The 'Papain' content is significant and the enzyme that helps in digesting proteins. It grows in abundance in India.

Now, the US, Mexico, and Puerto Rico are the biggest commercial producers of papaya in the world. Besides its papain content, it is also a rich source of antioxidant nutrients like carotenes, Vitamin C, Vitamin B, flavonoids, folate, minerals, potassium and magnesium, and fiber. Its pulp is also a core component for many facial creams, moisturizers, and shampoos. If you have never eaten it, then try this refreshingly sweet, tasty and exotic tropical fruit today. The best thing is that it is available all year long. Its seeds are also very useful. Herbalists give its seed powder to the children to kill parasites and bacteria in the digestive system. I call it 'delicious food' and some call it 'fruits of angels.' Clean and cut up one cup of papaya which is one serving. The best time to eat it is two hours after consuming meals.

Boosts Immunity: It is important to have a healthy immune system to fight against various infections. Eating a couple of servings every day can help boost your immunity and control your cravings the entire day. Because of its Vitamin C, it will also strengthen your immune system, and you may get fewer infections.

Lose Weight: If you want to lose weight, remember to add this beneficial fruit in your life and start losing weight. In India, if you join any Nature Cure Organization to lose weight or for any treatment, they will first advise you to eat papaya. The high fiber in it helps to push out the toxins from your body, eliminates constipation and helps lose weight. One medium papaya possesses 120 calories. Since it is filling, it will give a feeling of fullness and will also control the cravings.

Diabetics: Though papaya is sweet by nature, it is low in sugar and diabetic patients can enjoy it. The natural sweetness in it is not harmful to the diabetics. The high fiber and beneficial properties make papaya a super fruit for them.

Vision: This delicious fruit, rich in Vitamin A and beta-carotene, includes lutein which keeps the mucous membranes in our eyes healthy by safeguarding them from damage. Rich Vitamin A, it protects our eyes from macular degeneration that develops as we age in life. Papaya is also highly rich in carotenoids which we need for the health of the eyes health.

Lower Cholesterol: Because it contains high fiber, it safeguards against the build-up plaque which accumulated in the arteries. You all know too much cholesterol build-up can put a block in the arteries and lead to a heart attack, but regular consumption of this beautiful fruit helps keep the arteries open and healthy; thus lowering the cholesterol on a daily basis.

Heart Health: Natural Cure therapists recommend the consumption of this beneficial food for everyone to aid in having a healthy heart and avoid serious diseases like heart attacks.

Arthritis: Women, who eat a couple of servings of this food, have improved the health of their bones which helps reduces joint pain. Because it is high in anti-inflammatory properties that contain Vitamin C, it helps keep arthritis under control and one feels less uncomfortable. Just remember, it is good for your bones.

Improves Digestion: Papaya includes a digestive enzyme called papain which has high fiber, and that enhances digestion and cleanses the colon easily. When you eat heavy packaged foods or eat in restaurants, then papaya comes in to rescue your metabolism. Eating a cup of papaya two hours after consuming meals improves your digestive system.

Helps during Menstruation: Eating papaya regularly aids women in relieving menstrual pain and regulates and eases flow during periods. The enzyme papain contained in this fruit can calm menstrual pain if have many servings. It will also help in balancing hormonal levels as one grows.

It Is Anti-Aging: Who does not want to feel and look young? This fruit because of its high properties of Vitamin C, Vitamin E, and antioxidants such as beta-carotene, assists in protecting the skin from free radical damages, thus preventing fine lines and various signs of aging. For a beautiful skin tone, use papaya paste with honey and a pinch of sugar and massage gently on face, neck and hands keeping it on for 20 minutes. Rub again with wet hands for a few moments; wash it off and enjoy a silky soft and glowing skin. Repeat this process three times a week for great results.

Hair Health: Being a licensed aesthetician, I understand we need Vitamin A for healthy hair and scalp. Consuming papaya every day bringing Vitamin A into your body boosts the health of hair follicles, strengthens the hair, and enhances the growth of new hair. Blend papaya and onion with a little water; make a thin paste and apply to the scalp massaging with fingertips. Leave it on for 20 minutes and wash your hair with lukewarm water. Repeat this process twice a week and enjoy beautiful, silky, shiny and thick hair. You may eat two servings of papaya a day and live a healthy life

Reduce Stress: This excellent fruit is rich in numerous nutrients, such as Vitamin C, that help keep one free from stress and tension. I knew its benefits and sometimes, I used to take cut up papaya in a container to work as my lunch. Papaya's valuable properties help one to stay cool mentally and physically, and it can also aid in regulating stress. Herbalists always recommend this plant to people who suffer from anxiety and depression.

Prevent Cancer: Papaya is rich in antioxidants and flavonoids that protect body cells from cancer. the large quantity of beta-carotene in this fruit protects against colon and prostate cancer growth. It is a super food and also world's healthiest food

Soybean

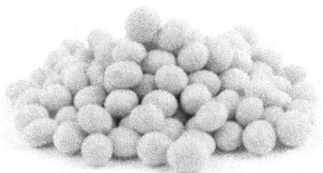

Soybeans are high in fat like protein. Except peanuts, most of the legumes contain between 2 to 14 percent fat, and soybeans contain 19 percent fat. Most of the fat in soybeans is unsaturated and useful. It is one of the few plants that contain Polyunsaturated, monounsaturated and saturated fats. The polyunsaturated fat content of soybean contains Omega-3 fatty acid. The omega–3 fats present in it makes soy uniquely healthy and nutritious. Omega-3 fatty acids are an essential nutrient which helps to reduce the risk of cancer and heart disease. Soybeans are the most alkaline food and help with acidity. Its products are available in the form of milk, flour, nuggets, granules, tofu, tempeh, miso, and cooked whole soybeans. In 1999, the FDA approved the heart health benefits of including at least 25 grams soy protein every day in a diet low in saturated fat and cholesterol.

Vitamins and Minerals: Since soy is a fat like protein, its foods are high in minerals and vitamins. It also includes potassium, folate, and fiber. Soy is attracting the attention of research scientists around the world for health properties and high nutrition values.

Cancers: Soy can lower risk of developing cancers such as breast, colon, and prostate. It can also protect against skin cancer.

Osteoporosis and Arthritis: Because of its high contents of fat it lubricates the joints thus reducing inflammation in the bones and reducing the pain in the joints. Besides helping in osteoporosis and arthritis condition, it also contributes to strengthening the bones. It possesses a good amount of Vitamin D and is rich in calcium in comparison to the commonly used legumes. Half a cup of tofu can include between 130 to 700 mg of calcium as per its processing methods, and one cup of soy milk possesses around 95 mg of calcium.

Diabetes: Diabetes has been on the rise in the global population for more than a decade. Soybeans are an effective method of prevention and management of this disease primarily because soybeans have shown an ability to increase insulin receptors in the body, thereby helping to manage the disease effectively or prevent it from occurring in the first place. Early studies focusing on this particular relationship of soy products to a decrease in Type 2 diabetes are still in the early stages, but the early results are very promising, primarily in Asian populations.

Sleep Disorders: Soybeans promote to regulate numerous aspects of the metabolism, which can aid in reducing sleep disorders and insomnia. However, it also has a high content of magnesium, which is a mineral content. It is directly increases the quality, extent, and rest and peaceful sleep.

Imbalanced Hormones: Regular consumption of half a cup of cooked soybeans five days a week can help to alleviate hot flashes associated with menopause.

Heart Health: We should plan our daily diet around a wide variety of nutritious soy foods like soy milk, tempeh, tofu, miso, and edamame. It is essential to add whole grains, fresh vegetables, fruits, and exercise. I want to remind my American folks to make healthier food choices and be smart about building a healthy plate at meals time. I will also emphasize vegetables, all greens, plant-based protein and dairy foods. This seed improves blood vessels such as real elasticity of artery walls and keeps them healthy.

For Pregnant Women: The vitamin B complex levels in soybeans are impressive as well, and the high levels of folic acid and Vitamin B complex are crucial for pregnant women. Including both the contents soybeans is a superb food. Folic acid content ensures the prevention of neural tube defects in infants that ensure a healthy baby.

Cholesterol: The effects of its protein help to lower cholesterol. In 1999, USDA came up with a health claim stating that 25 grams of soy protein per day may reduce the risk of heart disease. Most soy foods are also low in saturated and trans fats. This is the reason the American Heart Association has recognized soy foods as an overall heart-healthy diet.

Constipation: Because of its high fiber, soy helps to stimulate the digestive system and maintains regularity. Eating half a cup of cooked soybean for breakfast or lunch gives a feeling of fullness, and you do not munch all day.

Fiber: Soy is an excellent source of fiber. A serving of soybeans possesses approximately eight grams of dietary fiber. Processed foods such as soy milk and tofu include a tiny fiber, whereas, the foods that utilize the whole grain like soy flour, soy protein, soy sprouts, and tempeh contain high fiber. It is high in iron, but its protein reduces iron absorption. Iron is better absorbed from fermented soy foods such as miso, tempeh, and sprouts.

Works as Probiotics: Soy contains Vitamin B 12, calcium, selenium, magnesium, and all the amino acids essential to human health. This plant is rich in probiotics in the form of fermented soy products such as sprouts, tempeh, yogurt, and miso. Regular consumption of soy foods helps the human body to safeguard from harmful bacteria and live a healthy life. BUT IF YOU ARE SUFFERING FROM THYROID, THEN STAY AWAY FROM SOY BEANS.

NOTE: - It is a boon for the vegans.

Spinach

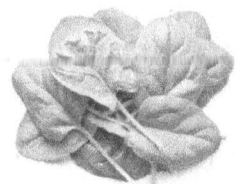

The delicate, bright, and vibrant-looking spinach leaves are full of nutrients, enzymes, minerals and vitamins. They are not only appealing to the eye but are also more nourishing. They look entirely alive and vital and have a high level of vitamin C. Its color is so appetizing that it compels me to pick up a bunch or a box whenever I am in a grocery store. Eating this plant frequently helps remove many light conditions in the body. Its supply of high vitamin C helps protect the body and the digestive system. These dark leafy green spinach are crucial for bone, hair and skin health and provide us protein, calcium, and iron.

Lowers Blood Pressure: It contains high potassium content and doctors recommend spinach to the individuals with high blood pressure. It helps to lower the effects of sodium in the body. Sometimes a low potassium intake can be a risk factor for developing high blood pressure. A high sodium intake can also result in water retention in the body, and your feet and legs may swell.

Bone health: There is a risk of bone fracture if a low consumption of vitamin K continues. Adequate vitamin K intake is essential for good health. It helps improve calcium absorption and can reduce urinary excretion of calcium.

Eliminate Constipation: It is high in fiber and water content, and these both contribute to cleansing the digestive tract and eliminate constipation. It also promotes a healthy colon and maintains regularity.

Healthy skin and hair: It possesses high vitamin A, which is important for sebum production to keep hair moisturized and hydrated. We need Vitamin A for the growth of our all bodily tissues, including skin and hair. All leafy greens including spinach are high in vitamin C and are vital for the building and maintenance of collagen, which provides structure to skin and hair. We all know iron-deficiency is a common cause of hair loss, and we can prevent it with adequate intake of iron-rich foods, like spinach; thus we see fewer wrinkles on our face.

Cancer Prevention: Spinach, leafy greens, and all green vegetables are full of chlorophyll which has proved to safeguard the effects at blocking the generation of cancer cells. For your information, grilling the foods at a high temperature also can generate cancer. With simple precautions and awareness, we all can avoid many physical conditions.

Asthma: Patients, who consume a high amount of certain nutrients have a lower risk to develop asthma. One of these nutrients is beta-carotene and spinach is an excellent source of it. Apricots, carrots, pumpkin, broccoli, cantaloupe, are also rich sources of beta-carotene.

When you buy vegetables and fruits, wash them thoroughly and juice them; no cooking involved. We call it a vital food and when you consume this kind of essential foods, every day you do not lose your vitality. In India, people with all sorts of different diseases, are cured with fresh juices.

Homemade fresh juice is delicious, light and pure and it assimilates in the blood stream quickly as you consume. It is also refreshing and filling. These fluids are considered alkaline food and we all should try to eat these kinds of foods as much as possible. This category of foods are very compatible with the human digestive system, but acidic food produces gas and creates problems in our body, which later turn into horrible diseases. All the green vegetables also come under the alkaline category of foods and are believed to be the best "internal cleanser" and "best alkaline body support." The human body is slightly alkaline with a pH of 7.4 level and chemical processes of the body function most efficiently in this condition. All the waste of our body is eliminated properly when the body functions proficiently. We should try to keep a balance of our intake of food and try to consume more alkaline food like soups, fruits, and vegetables, than acidic food.

When we consume more protein, it sits in the intestines and forms thin layers. It causes gas and fresh juice and a smoothie of leafy greens and vegetables, does the job of cleaning and scraping this foreign material from our system; thus enhancing our health to a better level.

While juicing or making a smoothie, add a handful of fresh spinach as it makes a potent drink. If one can handle this drink twice a day, one may gradually eliminate many physical ailments such as diabetes, skin disorders, and migraine.

Note: SPINACH CONTAINS A VERY HIGH CONTENT OF VITAMIN K. IF YOU ARE TAKING ANY MEDICATION FOR A HEART PROBLEM LIKE WARFARIN OR CUMEDIN, PLEASE CONSULT YOUR DOCTOR BEFORE YOU START EATING SPINACH OR ANY OTHER VEGETABLE.

Sweet Basil (Tulsi)

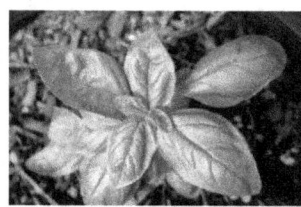

You may be using sweet basil only for cooking, but it can do much more if you know its benefits and the methods to use. We are all aware its culinary uses but today you will discover its advantages and bring it to your day-to-day life to enjoy living better naturally. It is a famous herb recognized by the Ayurvedic practitioners, and they believe in this herb and call it an 'all cure remedy.' In India, the Nature Cure therapists encourage people to grow basil at home and use it lavishly because it helps heal many mental and physical conditions.

Pesto Basil: The first thing that comes to mind is the most popular basil pesto. We all like it, enjoy mixed in our salads, raw vegetables, and especially on toast with butter. It is the most modern use with variations in different cultures around the world, but it is the best way to consume it.

Blood sugar: There is some evidence that basil can help level out blood sugar if regularly consumed as a juice or tea.

Helps Stress: Most herbalists suggest that one boil two cups of sweet basil leaves in three cups of water for a couple of minutes then add to a warm bath to help the reduction of stress and enjoyment to relaxation.

A Tonic Drink: Chew five leaves of basil every morning and swallow with a glass of water or take one teaspoonful of fresh basil juice in the same quantity of water early morning. It helps your body produce more energy and feel secure. Regular consumption of this mixer also helps strengthen muscles and bones.

Liver: If you boil a quarter cup of its leaves in a glass of water for five minutes, cool it, strain it and drink it every day. It will help an enlarged liver shrink and also relieve the liver's other problems.

Cooking: You can use fresh or dried basil frequently in any dish. In salads, it increases the taste and the flavor. Basil is used a lot in many different cuisines around the world. It adds a unique flavor that you get only from this herb. Sometimes, I use this plant in my curries when I invite my Italian friends. My Nature Cure teacher always advised us to drink basil tea instead of regular tea because basil tea relieves gas and regular tea generates gas. You just boil basil leaves in water for one minute, strain it, add a teaspoon of honey and enjoy.

Calming Effects: A cup of basil tea always creates a calming impact on the mind. If you soak its dried leaves overnight and drink the water next day, it assists in calming down the stomach and often helps soothe indigestion and alleviate the feelings of being bloated.

Fainting: If someone faints, grind its leaves with a pinch of salt and put some drops in the nose. The person will be revealed to her/his senses pretty soon.

Coughing and Common Colds: Long ago when I lived in India, I saw that many women had a basil plant in the house. They boiled basil leaves and gave them to the children and even the adults in the family when they had a fever or were suffering from a cold or the flu. They believed its leaves calmed down a cough and fever. Also, they wrapped some dried leaves and put them under their pillows. I think its aroma also helps.

For A Headache: A facial steam using fresh or dried basil leaves can help alleviate a headache. Add a tablespoon of dried or a quarter cup of fresh basil leaf to 2 cups of boiling water in a medium pot. Turn the heat to medium, lean over the pot carefully, covering your head with a towel and breathe in the steam for 10-12 minutes until a headache starts to decrease. You will also get to experience the aroma of this 'great' plant throughout the house all day long.

Antibiotic properties: According to Ayurvedic Specialists, scientists are doing research and investigating the use of basil oil as a treatment for antibiotic resistant infections. Because of its antibiotic and antioxidant compounds, people are getting great healings, and it has become popular herb.

Insect Bites and Stings: If you are working outside in the back yard and an insect bites or stings you; immediately start chewing up basil leaves and rubbing crushed leaves on it if you do not have its oil at home. It will help relieve the pain and push insect's poisonous effect through waste.

Hiccups: If you are experiencing hiccups, mix one tablespoon of basil juice with one teaspoon of honey and eat slowly. They will disappear!

Ear Infections: Apart from eating this plant, herbalists also recommend using the oil in the ear to get rid of infections or other ear problems. This oil is antibacterial, and it works well.

Nose and Private Parts: If there is a pain in your nose or private parts for any reason, then take a handful of dried basil leaves and put them in a thin handkerchief, tie it and make a ball. Smell it as much as you can and the pain and ailment will slowly vanish.

I had a couple of basil plants in my back yard, and I used them lavishly in some dishes, but my family could not handle its aroma and pungency in every dish. I also used it a lot in my herbal tea. I dried it, and I am still using it. I suggest that everyone use it in any way they like. It is full of great benefits which are why it is called the 'All Cure' herb.

Sweet Potato

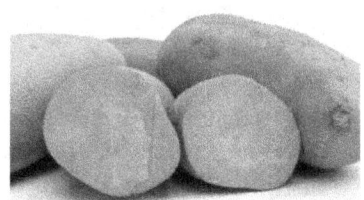

Sweet potatoes are always available everywhere. They are inexpensive; can be boiled, roasted, fried, and they are delicious. They have an unending list of benefits for health. They are high in fiber. I have only to say, cook the way you like but eat every day to stay healthy, young and beautiful. They possess beautiful orange, yellow, and red pigments, and experts call them carotenoids and are present in many plants. Carotenoids act as antioxidants within our bodies protecting against cellular damage and the effects of aging and even some chronic diseases. We can get these benefits only by eating certain foods.

Skin Health: They are high in Vitamin B6, and Vitamin B6 contributes to reducing the chemicals Homocysteine, which consumed in medicines, or products we eat, or the body produces. These compounds have harmful effects on our bodies such as degenerative diseases, including heart attacks, diabetes, or overweight. They are rich in Vitamin C, and we all know how this vitamin is essential to ward off common colds and flu! Vitamin C is also a crucial vitamin that promotes to strengthening our bones, tooth formation, stimulates digestion, and cell blood formation; helps to heal wounds faster, produces collagen and helps maintain skin's youthful elasticity. There are fewer wrinkles on the face. There is a contribution to coping with stress and protecting the body against toxins.

Heart Health: Regular consumption of this vegetable helps eliminate chemicals in our body, leaving us with a fewer physical disorders, especially heart health. It is rich in Magnesium that promotes a healthy heart, bones, muscles, blood and normal arteries. When human body has no disease, the heart is happy and does a fantastic job. The healthy heart keeps your body in good shape. It is a good carb, and we can consume it on a daily basis. I believe, it is better than eating wheat, and bread each day.

Immune System: Sweet potatoes possess iron. We all need this mineral to have sufficient energy in the body. Iron also plays many other important roles in our body, including the production of red and white blood and cells, resistance to fight stress and disease, effective for immune functioning, and the proper distribution of protein for a healthy metabolism. Active immune system or healthy metabolism is the second name of enjoying excellent health.

Constipation: If you regularly consume this vegetable, it promotes to clean the intestines, eliminate constipation and maintains regularity. You may steam it, cook with onions, mash it like potatoes and mix ingredients of your choice, puree it, or bake it, roast it or grill it; it comes out delicious. I eat a large piece of sweet potato; do not care for bread, and enjoy my lunch with good carbs. It is filling, nutritious, delicious, and enables a natural bowel movement.

Stress: Sweet potatoes are an excellent source of magnesium, which is a relaxation and anti-stress mineral. Magnesium is necessary for healthy artery, blood, bone, heart, muscle, and nerve function. Experts estimate that approximately 80 percent of the population in North America may be deficient in this important mineral.

Relaxes Muscles and protects Kidneys: This vegetable is a source of potassium and carries one of the essential electrolytes that can promote heartbeat and nerve signals. Potassium performs a regular variety of important functions, such as reducing swelling, relaxing the muscles, and protecting and controlling the activity of the kidneys.

Diabetics: Sweet potatoes have a natural sweetness in it. The simple sugars assimilate into the bloodstream gradually, helping the diabetic patient feel an increased and balanced energy. Being a natural sugar, the body accepts it happily, and there is no fear of gaining Good weight. If you cook it adding more sugar to it, there are chances of weight gain.

Good For Eyes: The color of sweet potatoes shows us they are full of carotenoids like beta carotene. Beta carotene, which is Vitamin A, is excellent for our eye health. It strengthens and brightens our eyes, and helps decrease the eye problems. Carotenoids are potent antioxidants that strengthen the immune system; boost men's vitality, and fight against cancer. If we consume food rich in carotenoids and beta carotene, there may be fewer diseases in our bodies.

Tomato

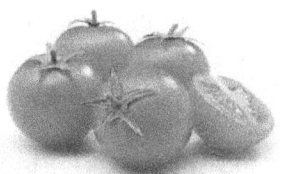

Sometimes we compliment someone and often say, "Your cheeks look like tomatoes" that is when someone is in excellent health. Ripe and juicy tomatoes are a great health benefit, always have a convertible bond in your mind. Did you ever imagine that the omnipresent tomato is a powerful agent of nutritional benefits? We, in Nature Cure, believe tomato is a fruit as well as a vegetable and we use it extensively in preparing a large variety of dishes. Tomato is a naturally rich source of protein; that is good for muscle building and cell repair. Tomatoes and its products have the ability to contribute to the skin to absorption, oxygen that helps prevents age spots and several signs of aging. It is an excellent means to provide us an amazing natural skin treatment. It aids the skin to look healthy, beautiful and younger with little effort.

The Powerhouse of Nutrients: According to the USDA, tomatoes include all the potent specific nutrients needed for proper functioning of the human body. It provides approximately 20% of the daily vitamin intake per serving, which we require each day.

Cooking: People use the tomato in vegetarian and non-vegetarian dishes all over the world and also for snacks. The most famous pizzas, salads, sandwiches, and cocktails we make with tomatoes, and you could say without tomatoes these foods would be incomplete and tasteless. It is the world's best food and makes delicious dishes.

A Fruit: Being a favorite of the herbalists, they recommend consuming the tomato raw like fruit for the best result. We can eat a fresh tomato like fruit, grill it, steam and cook it with any dish of your choice. This plant is full of numerous nutritional benefits and is highly popular in many cultures. My Natural Cure Teacher always said in class, "Eat one tomato every day for breakfast and you will have cheeks like a tomato."

Filling Food: Vegetables are full of water and because of their water content, they give you feeling of fullness, moisturizes the skin and keeps it healthy and looking fresh. Tomatoes also include a good amount of fiber that also aids in feeling full.

Heart Health: This fruit is highly rich in potassium content and carries a high level of potassium. It contributes to control of heart rate and is very helpful in preventing heart diseases and strokes. Tomatoes also contain necessary nutrients, such as niacin, folate, and vitamin B6, that also contribute to the reduction of heart disease risk.

Eyes: Tomatoes possess Vitamin A, Flavonoid B complex, folate and thiamine and many other nutrients that contribute to cure skin and eye disorders naturally.

Lowers Blood Pressure: They include potent minerals and nutrients that assist in protecting the body from High Cholesterol and High Blood Pressure.

Teeth and Bones: Tomato, being rich in Calcium, promotes strengthening the bones and bone formation in the human body and also supports in maintaining teeth in a healthy state.

Constipation: We all know tomato includes flavonoid antioxidants, such as lycopene. Mix two tablespoons of tomato paste in 12 oz. of water with a spoon of olive oil and drink early morning; it helps prevents hemorrhoids, weight loss and elimination of constipation is a proven fact. Eating one large tomato for breakfast, stimulates the digestive system and pushes out toxins through the waste, maintaining regularity.

Helps Cancer: The flavonoid antioxidants in this vegetable also contribute to preventing certain unwanted eruptions in the body, reactions in the lungs, colon, and breasts that can lead to cancer. These antioxidants assist in the treatment of cancer by preventing cancer cells in the body. These compounds also help to stop by blocking free radicals from happening any further.

Acne and Rash: Vitamin A and C are commonly found in many acne treating medicines and ointments. The high acidic content in tomatoes helps to treat rashes and acne. You may cut a tomato and rub frequently every day on the areas where you get a rash and after three weeks, the discoloration and the itch may also disappear.

Prevent Excess Oil: When I was studying Natural Cure, yoga, and meditation, my teacher showed the whole class as practical use 'To prevent excess oil secretion from the face.' Squeeze a small tomato in your hand and add one tablespoon of cucumber juice, apply to the face, and rub in gently with upward strokes. Leave on your face for 20 minutes and, then wash it off. This procedure helps remove the excess sebum production from your face that leads to clogging of the pores, and that leads to pimples, dirt builds up and uneven skin tone.

Signs of Ageing: In Natural Cure, we believe the tomato helps to slow our age and preventing fine lines and wrinkles. The lycopene is an excellent property of this fruit that makes a natural amazing anti-ageing product. Eating tomatoes and applying topical ingredients show significant results, and are very inexpensive compared to packaged cosmetic products.

Bleach Skin Naturally: Ayurvedic practitioners believe the tomato is a natural bleaching product. You can prepare a face pack by mixing two tablespoons of tomato pulp, one tablespoon of yogurt, and one tablespoon of oatmeal into a course powder. Apply to your face, neck and hands with a little massage and leave it on for 20 minutes. Before washing, press again gently with wet hands and wash it off. This combination of tomato pulp, oatmeal, and yogurt is very beneficial for the skin. If you apply this homemade pack on your face three days a week, it will contribute to a beautiful, soft and brighter skin.

Stress: Did you know big business are using tomato extract in luxurious body massage oils to safeguard and fight visible stress signs on the skin? These companies are also combining tomato extract with other essential ingredients and using it, in their eye creams. Eyes will look fresh and revitalized and will not show any stress signs.

Makes Perfect Astringent: You mash a quarter of an avocado with half of a fresh tomato. Apply the pulp to your face, neck and hands and massage gently. Leave on for 20 minutes. Before washing, again rub gently with wet hands and slide on your skin. This procedure will make your skin look so smooth, soft and moisturized. You may also experience your skin cleansed thoroughly with a glowing complexion.

Fight Cellular Damage: If you consume two tablespoons of tomato paste daily first thing in the early morning; it can do wonders for you. Because of its antioxidants and lycopene, it contributes to longevity, safeguards against cellular damage, and the reddening of your skin. It helps to reduce free radicals from the body, eliminate constipation; restore moisture and give you a youthful skin.

Prevents Sunburn: As per Prevention Magazine, if you consume five tablespoons of tomato paste daily for three consecutive months, you are naturally protected from sunburn. You can also treat sun burnt skin by applying fresh squeezed tomato juice in the affected areas.

Cooling Effect: Tomato has a cooling effect. If you use a pack with tomato and yogurt on the hands and under the feet; keep it covered with plastic wrap and wash it off after 20 minutes. Both ingredients have a cooling effect, and you may get a boost to making the skin moisturized soft and supple.

Smooth And Glowing Face: Squeeze a little tomato in your hand, add half a teaspoon of honey and apply on your face. After 20 minutes wash it off and witness a smooth and glowing skin.

Remove Dead Skin: Mix one tablespoon of fresh tomato juice with half a teaspoon of sugar. Apply on the face; massage gently in circular motions and wash it off after 10 minutes. It sloughs off the dead cells on the skin and gives you a feeling of clean and fresh looking skin. You may also cut one tomato into two halves and sprinkle some sugar over it, and gently massage face with it. It also helps to remove dead cells to get a clean looking skin.

NOTE: - Though tomato is high in antioxidants, minerals and vitamins, it also includes Vitamin K that can interrupt your medicine if you are taking heart medication like Warfarin. Before eating a tomato or starting to eat any fruit or vegetable, please consult with your doctor.

Turmeric

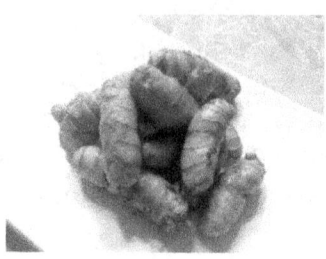

Turmeric is a very beneficial herb. You may also call it a spice.
It grows like ginger and potatoes under the soil. It is widely grown all over India. It looks like ginger, but smaller and thinner in size. It comes from the ginger family. It looks orange when peeled, but mostly it is dried and ground into powder. While grinding a few drops of oil are added so it does not scatter. After drying, it looks yellow, and this is the reason it is called yellow turmeric. I call it a miracle healer from the kitchen. It is also known as Curcuma Longa in Latin. It is the only spice several scientists have researched for its medical properties and ancient remedies. Now findings tell us turmeric can heal any disease. This root helps to cleanse the body and is used as a preventive to always stay healthy. I use fresh turmeric as a Pro-biotic.

Turmeric, in India, is a common spice and is utilized by each family in everyday cooking. Here in the US, Indian communities use turmeric every day and it is always available in my kitchen. As per our ancient scriptures, this root of golden yellow turmeric has been used as a spice and for medical purposes for over 6,000 years in the treatment of pains and aches, skin diseases, cuts and open wounds, and common colds. It is also used as a blood purifier and as a cleansing of a urinal track.

It has been one of the most ancient remedies like ginger and garlic. Even now in modern time, I believe that 70% of the people of India, who live in villages and small towns, still use turmeric for many ailments. I remember when we were little, if my brother would come home with some blood on his leg or foot, my mom used to scoop out turmeric powder from the kitchen, put on the wound and press it down with her thumb for a minute. Later when the blood stopped, she would put more turmeric, a piece of cotton and would bandage it.

There are several Naturopaths and Ayurvedic doctors in India, who treat people with herbs, spices, yoga, pranayam and meditation in the villages as well as in the major cities like New Delhi, Mumbai, Bangalore, and Chennai. In fact, many Bollywood and Hollywood celebrities, high-level business people and dignitaries, now prefer to go to Nature Cure doctors for their mental and physical problems because they are sick and tired of available injurious drugs and doctors who have just one aim, that of minting money without having a relationship with the patients. In most of the villages, there are no medical professionals available, but there are Hakeem, who are popular for their Natural Healing methods and remedies. The public trusts them because they get cured.

Turmeric root is so beneficial we can use it regularly, to help ourselves as a preventative to help ourselves against horrible disorders like influenza, colds, virus, allergies, arthritic pain, Alzheimer's disease, heart and urinal tract problems, and cancer, while detoxifying the body.

I buy a quarter pound of raw turmeric root and wash it thoroughly with a brush. I make a paste in the blender with 2 oz. of water, bottle and refrigerate it. I swallow half a teaspoon of this paste first thing in the morning and avoid getting sick. Let me tell you, winter is approaching, and it brings allergies and many unpleasant problems with it, and you do not want to suffer. Its taste is neither bitter, sour nor tangy. It is not peppery hot. In fact, it is bland and a little pungent.

For more information, you may read 'TURMERIC The Golden Wonder Herb,' an excellent book by Taryn Forrelli ND. The other name I found is TURMERIC: 'The Ayurvedic Spice of Life' written by Prashanti de Jager MS, which tells us in detail what a wonderful herb turmeric is.

Turnip

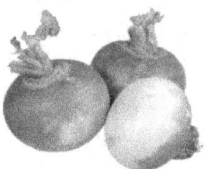

Like most other vegetables, Turnips are low in calories like most other vegetables. They are quite nutritious. In India, they are for human consumption, but at some places, they are given to farm animals. They possess a variety of significant health benefits. One has to know the knack, 'How to cook it,' honestly speaking; it is delicious. High fiber diets have been found to absorb more water thus making the bowel movement very smooth. One cup of cooked turnips provides 4 grams of fiber. It is world's healthiest food. Select vegetables that are small and thick in size. Small plants have a sweet and mild flavor. Choose with green tops that have bright color and look fresh. You can use in cooking or add to your salads. My Nature Cure teacher always said, "You do not need a calcium supplement, just eat turnips and feel healthy and safe." Ayurvedic practitioners call it 'healer of common ailments.'

Prevent Cancer: The vegetables, which include cruciferous, are high with phytochemicals and antioxidants levels. Turnip also contains these compounds that contribute to reducing the risk of cancer. The essential compounds that appear in it help prevent and reduce the effects of cancer. These are the plants that bear natural chemicals that break into different compounds while digesting it; promote the liver process toxins, fight the effects of carcinogens and can hinder the growth of the tumor cells. If we include turnip dish or eat this uncooked vegetable in our daily diet that can reduce the risk of rectal tumors, breast, and colon cancer. Any vegetable, which tastes a little bitter or pungent, gives them the cancer-fighting power.

Help Lower Blood Pressure: The foods containing high dietary fiber such as turnips and broccoli have shown to have multiple benefits for reducing blood pressure and protecting the heart. A healthy diet with fruits and vegetables has shown positive results in lowering the blood pressure. Turnips include potassium, which contributes to bringing blood pressure down by releasing sodium out of the body.

Lose Weight And Detoxify The System: Turnips and other cruciferous vegetables that are full of fiber contribute to keeping you full longer and are low in calories. You do not munch the whole day. Consuming fiber-rich food keeps blood sugar stable and detoxifies the system. The turnips are rich in fiber that encourages drinking more water, and the result is you do not suffer from constipation. You enjoy a healthy digestive tract; promote regularity and helps you lose some pounds. Turnips are low in calories and can incorporate into your daily meals as an effective weight loss program. Their valuable fiber content aids regulate metabolism, safeguards body mass and support a healthy and active colon.

Maintain Vision: For good vision, an adequate Vitamin C intake is crucial and vegetable like turnip, provide us increased protection against the UV light damage. We think of lemon or grapefruit when we talk about Vitamin C, but there are lots of fruits and vegetables that possess surprisingly high content of Vitamin C. Turnip is also great with this compound and can help to maintain our vision if we eat two turnips a day. Some individuals believe in a higher intake of fruits and vegetables (4 servings a day) that promotes decrease the risk of eye problems like macular degeneration and makes their eyes healthier.

Bone Health: Turnip is a primary source of calcium and potassium, which are crucial for healthy bones, their growth, and maintenance. If you regularly consume turnip, it safeguards the joint damage, risk of starting osteoporosis problem and the Arthritis pains. It is full of nutrients, rich in fiber, an excellent source of calcium, mineral, and enzymes that strengthen the bones and support the body's production of connective tissues. Because of its significant anti-inflammatory properties and a large amount of Vitamin K, it helps in preventing heart attacks, heart strokes and reduces the inflammation of the joints; thus keeping them healthy. But if you have a heart condition and you are taking medicine Warfarin, and then check with your doctor.

Help Lung Health: The individuals, who smoke; suffer from Vitamin A deficiency, resulting in lung inflammation, short breathing, heavy breathing, and other lung conditions. Vitamin A present in turnips contributes to maintaining healthy lungs by fighting against the defects.

Cure Asthma: The anti-inflammatory properties and its pungency promote to fight asthma condition and contribute to a little ease in breathing. We know turnips by their high content of vitamin C, which is the powerhouse of antioxidants. These exceptional properties are very efficient in helping to heal an asthma patient and decreasing the symptoms of asthma. The Studies have already shown proofs of feeding turnips (cooked and raw) to asthmatic patients and aiding to less wheezing.

Healer of Common Ailments: The great healing power of this vegetable is very useful in safeguarding many common ailments. Regular consumption of this vegetable (cooked or raw) can aid to decrease constipation, hemorrhoids and lack of hunger and it can also help flush out kidney stones if they are small enough.

Water

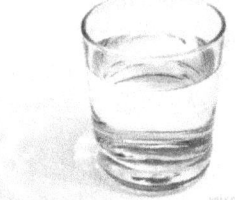

Water is FREE! It is available in abundance. Feel free to drink water as much as your body requires. Drink it to your health, because your body cries for water. You can choose bottled water or filtered water, you need to have belief in me; it is still cheaper than those with high sugar and fat-filled latte. It is an excellent moisturizer, and a wonderful cleanser that keeps your body hydrated and bones lubricated. Drinking one and a half liter of water first thing in the early morning helps individuals suffering from hemorrhoids, indigestion, to push out the toxins from your system. Diabetes, gas trapped in the stomach, weight loss and skin problems, and sleeping well, and much more are other benefits. In Yoga, we call it "Usha Paan;" it is a Yoga Kriya, and here in the USA, medical professionals call it "Aqua Therapy."

Flush Out Toxins: Water is a wonderful exfoliate and an excellent moisturizer for your skin. It flushes out the toxins from your body, keeping the system clean and healthy. Water aids the digestive system to get rid of waste through sweat and reduces the risk of kidney stones and UTI problem. I have seen people terribly suffering from this disease, and if you are a water guzzler, you may never face this UTI (urinary tract infections) as a problem. I will say you are not sick; you are thirsty! Quench your thirst with water, not with medicines and chemicals.

Aging Slow: Water is an excellent cleanser of the digestive system and naturally detoxifies the human body. It helps maintain your skin soft, fresh, smooth, and glowing and helps prevent the formation of pimples. Your face gets rid of fine lines. In Nature Cure, we call water "The best anti-aging agent!"

Look Young: Water is an amazing natural treatment for the human body. It has numerous benefits for the skin and digestive system. It helps replenish your skin and detoxifies your digestive track. It also promotes to tone the skin, clears and tighten the pores and show a fewer fine lines on the face. The potassium content in lemon helps nourish brain and nerve cells

Lose Weight: When you drink enough water that your body requires on a daily basis, It feels happy, make you more alert; think better and boosts your energy. It also helps decrease by-products of fat and assists you to eat an adequate portion of food. Individuals, who intend to lose weight; may drink a full cup of water before they eat or drink anything so that their stomach feels full and do not munch the whole day. Remember, water stimulates your metabolism, it is a natural appetite suppressant and has no calories. If you drink a tall glass of lukewarm water with juice of half a lemon and a quarter teaspoon of sea salt in the morning, it promotes lose weight.

Boost Energy: Our brain is mostly water and drinking enough of it, helps you think, focus and concentrate better. It also increases your energy levels, and you feel less fatigued. Especially, when you drink a full glass of water before and after a workout, the brain purifies, nourishes it, and the nerve cells.

Constipation: Water is an essential agent for the digestion tract. It aids in digesting the food and safeguards against constipation. Constipation is the primary cause of all horrible diseases, and I call it 'a physical disorder of wealthy society.' Drinking one and a half liter of water first thing in the early morning helps individuals suffering from hemorrhoids, indigestion, diabetes, gas trapped in the stomach, to lose weight, skin problems and much more. In Yoga, we call it "Usha Paan;" it is a Yoga Kriya, and here in the USA, medical professionals call it "Aqua Therapy."

Boosts Immune System: If you are a water guzzler, you are a very healthy person, and there are fewer chances to get sick. It stimulates your metabolism and fights against minor ailments like flu, headaches and colds. May you feel healthy most of the time? My Nature Cure teacher told me that the water even helps to the heart patients if they drink a lot of water.

Natural Headache Remedy: Next time, if you have a severe headache, drink a full glass of water every hour. You only have to go to the bathroom frequently, but it aids to eliminate a problem. Water helps to balance to maintain the pH Level in the body and contributes to relieve headaches, which are mostly caused by dehydration. If you drink plenty of water regularly, there are chances you may not get one.

Arthritis And Inflammation: Water helps dissolve uric acid from the bones and joints that promote to reduce pain and inflammation in joints and knees. It is a free and simple treatment to stay healthy if one drinks plenty of water every day. When your body lubricates, it functions at its best, and you feel healthy and happy. Proper hydration contributes to keeping joints lubricated, and muscles are more elastic that make our joints painless. Back home in India, my mom taught us to drink a glass of water before we leave home and when we come back; sit, relax, and drink a glass of water because it is a life boosting element.

Note: - To cure body with water, read an excellent book on water authored by Dr. F. Batmanghelidj, M.D.

Watermelon

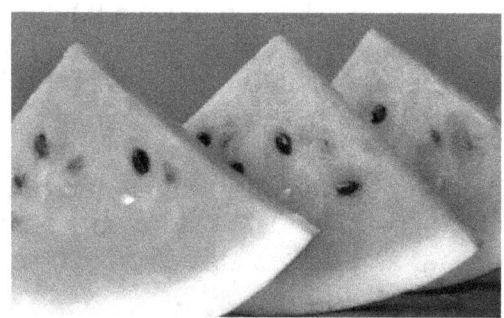

Most of us have the traditional belief watermelon is made up of only water and sugar, but it is a dense food with a combination of nutrients, has a high amount of antioxidants, it provides numerous vitamins and minerals and has a small amount of calories. It includes natural sweetness which our body absorbs quickly and is beneficial for our body. Watermelon has become familiar with the summer season, picnics, and parties for good reasons. It has a hydrating quality, sweet taste, refreshing in the heat and also provides a guilt-free, low maintenance dessert for kids and adults. We all enjoy it and it is also inexpensive. It comes from the family of cantaloupe and honeydew. You can find five types of watermelons in the market: seeded, seedless, mini (we also call it as personal), orange and yellow. They were always in a round shape, but Japan has invented square watermelons which look funny but are easy to slice and have the same taste.

Maintain Collagen And Firm Skin: One cup of watermelon possesses 21% of our daily need of Vitamin C intake. In fact, the human body requires this adequate amount of Vitamin C for the building and maintenance of collagen, which helps provide structure to skin and hair. This fruit also contributes to overall hydration, which is essential for having healthy looking firm skin and lustrous hair. It helps us look young.

Pregnancy: Most doctors recommend healthy and rich foods for pregnant women and watermelon, being rich in antioxidant compounds, vitamins, nutrients, minerals, and enzymes is one of the best foods to keep them full and healthy. Sinoc it contains water and natural sugars; it is a light food, digests quickly, boosts energy, and does not contribute to gaining weight. Pregnant women need strength and they can afford to eat this fruit a slice at a time throughout the day to help them stay active and stress-free.

Prevent Asthma: People who consume a high amount of certain nutrients have a lower risk of developing asthmatic conditions. This plant contains Vitamin C which is available in many fruits and vegetables including watermelon.

Lose Weight: Eating lots of vegetables and fruits of all kinds has a long association with a reduced risk of many lifestyle-related health conditions. Many studies have shown that increasing consumption of plant-based foods like watermelons decrease the risk of obesity, diabetes, heart disease, overall mortality and contributes to a healthy complexion, thick hair, increased energy, and weight loss.

Blood Pressure and Heart: This fruit also helps lower blood pressure. A study by the American Journal of Hypertension shows that watermelon extract supplements reduced ankle blood pressure which is mostly seen in obese middle-aged adults with pre-hypertension or stage one hypertension. Its extract supplements improved arterial function. Diets rich in lycopene can also assist in protection against heart conditions

Cancer: The lycopene in watermelon is an excellent source of the high antioxidant Vitamin C and other antioxidants, which can aid in fighting the formation of free radicals known to generate cancer. In numerous studies the consumption of lycopene has shown good results in decreasing the risk of prostate and colon cancer.

Maintains Regularity: Watermelon, because of its water and fiber content, helps to prevent constipation and promotes regularity which results in a healthy digestive tract.

Hydration: This fruit contains 92% water and is full of essential electrolytes that our body needs. Watermelon is a great snack to have on hand in your refrigerator during the hot summer months to prevent dehydration. It is filling, refreshing, replenishing, satisfying and tasty. Just wash, slice, and store it in a plastic container in the refrigerator. Enjoy this tempting snack the whole day, one slice at a time.

Inflammation: As we all know, watermelon contains Choline which is a vital and versatile nutrient that assists the body in sleeping, muscle movement, remembering, learning and memory. Choline also contributes to maintaining the structure of cellular membranes, aids in the transmission of nerve impulses, helps in the absorption of fat in the digestive system and reduces chronic inflammation, thus easing pain in joints and body.

Sore Muscles: Watermelon is full of nutrients, and its juice has been shown to decrease muscle soreness and improve recovery time following exercise in athletes. It is due to the amino acids that watermelon contains. It may amaze you to know that I have seen people drinking its juice then rubbing a little bit on the sore muscle.

Hair and Nails: This fruit is also excellent for our skin because it contains a nutrient required for sebum production and contains Vitamin A that keeps hair moisturized. We all need Vitamin A for the growth of all body tissues, including skin and hair.

Yogurt

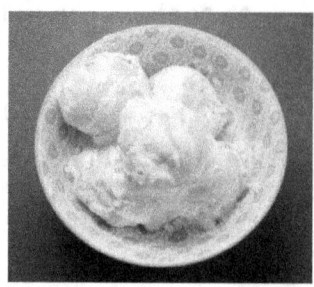

Yogurt is high in protein and is a powerhouse of bone-building calcium. It also promotes weight loss and keeps you healthy. Its protein and calcium are natural which digest quickly and faster, keeping our metabolism active and healthy. Half a cup of simple plain yogurt can give you enough protein and calcium for a day. Why did I use the words 'pure' and 'plain' yogurt? I make yogurt at home twice a week and believe me; it is 100% pure with no chemicals and no preservatives. When you buy it from the market, it includes salt, sugar, chemicals, thickening agent, and preservatives, but when I make it at home, it is only pure milk and is so easy to make. If we add a spoon of brown sugar or honey to our yogurt, it becomes more beneficial.

Loaded With Vitamins: In Nature Cure we believe, half a cup of yogurt (about 4-5 oz) makes one serving and is a significant source of Vitamin B5, Vitamin B12, potassium, phosphorous, zinc, iodine, and riboflavin. Vitamin B12 is mostly available in animal products, but people like me, who are vegetarian and do not consume even eggs or fish, get our best nutrients easily from yogurt. Vitamin B12 is an essential compound which maintains red blood cells and helps keep our nervous system functioning properly. We eat yogurt every day for lunch. Sometimes we add honey and on other occasions, we use a pinch of salt and pepper. We cook many dishes with yogurt. We make raita in a large variety, lassi (a drink with yogurt), sweet lassi, salty lassi, sweet creamy and delicious lassi, replenishing mango lassi, avocado smoothie, and many more things and we try to eat a couple of servings daily. Eating more yogurt encourages us to stay healthy and vibrant.

Flatten Abs: If you want flat abs, choose to eat yogurt, at least, three times a day. If you fast and live on yogurt, you may also consume green leaves; as you need lots of fiber, for your system and you will experience how your stomach starts melting fat. Remember; exercise is the keyword to lose weight and if you do not move your body you are giving too must rest to your body. You may stick to a 6-7 oz. serving three times a day with appropriate exercise and enjoy the great results. Do you know that the accumulated fat around your waist produces the cortisol hormone which encourages your system to build up, even more, belly fat? While eating yogurt; the calcium signals the fat cells to push out cortisol, making it a little easier for us to drop some weight while at the same time, the amino acids promote the burning of fat.

Good Bacteria: We eat yogurt as probiotics; it means it can fight infections. People swallow probiotic capsules and tablets, but we, instead eat yogurt. When you buy it from the market, it says "live and active cultures," which means the yogurt contains good bacteria or probiotics and is very beneficial for the intestines. This good bacteria lives in the digestive tract which contributes to destroying and pushing out bad, harmful bacteria that can generate intestinal infections.

Boosts energy after a workout: I used to drink half of a big tumbler (32 oz.) with a cup of homemade plain yogurt churned with water, we call it lassi, before going for a workout and the other half of it after the session and I always felt energized. It's high protein, good carbs, and calcium made an excellent session snack before and after the exercise. The one, half I drank before the exercise, energized me really and the half I took after the workout, cooled me down which improved hydration, and made me feel very relaxed. Also, the natural protein provides the amino acids which repair and strengthen muscles.

Homemade Pure yogurt: Homemade yogurt is the best; 100% pure with no added salt, sugar, or preservatives. It has its own sweet and creamy taste, and it is so cheap and easy to make, one can make it every day. It includes natural protein and calcium, but the one you buy from the market is very expensive and contains salt, sugar, and chemicals. Please read the label!

Lower Blood Pressure: Most of us eat more than twice the recommended amount of salt which is unhealthy. Overeating salt can lead to high blood pressure, hypertension, kidney and heart disease. The potassium, good content in yogurt, can help flush the excess sodium out of your body if you regularly eat yogurt. In fact, if you want to lower your blood pressure, start regular consumption, 2-3 servings daily of low-fat yogurt and yogurt lassi (yogurt drink) and amaze yourself with the exciting results.

Common Cold and Allergies: In Nature Cure, we believe regular consumption of half a cup of yogurt at breakfast can help you stay allergy-free in the changing seasons. Those eating 2-3 servings every day have much stronger and many more active helper T cells, which fight illness and infection than they did before they started consuming it. Because of its great benefits and good bacteria, yogurt contributes to sending signals to the immune-boosting cells in the body to empower and fight against harmful bacteria. People who suffer from allergies, especially who have weak resistant power, can also boost by adding yogurt to their meals. The individuals who consumed more than half a cup of it daily had fewer symptoms of cold and allergies because yogurt strengthens immunity and increases resistant power.

Dandruff: Mix a big pinch of salt in a quarter cup of yogurt and rub on the scalp. Leave it in for 20 minutes and wash it off. Dandruff will disappear entirely after three applications. If you mix juice from half a lemon in a quarter cup of yogurt, rub into hair and wash after 20 minutes, your hair will become healthy and stay dark naturally. And, if you mix with a big pinch of black pepper, rub on the scalp, leave in for 20 minutes and wash it off, you will enjoy silky, shiny, healthy hair.

Face and Skin: You can make many different kinds of face packs with this miracle dairy product and get the beautiful skin. When I had my babies, I applied yogurt on their tiny bodies, massaged gently and bathed them with lukewarm water for the first whole year. You may make a pack with yogurt and lemon, a pinch of sugar, or honey and course ground oats, or mustard oil and lemon; apply on your face, neck, and hands and massage gently. Let it dry. Again rub gently with wet fingertips in small circles and wash it off. After three weeks you can feel and see silky, soft and brighter skin.

Helps Maintain Your Smile: Though it has its natural sweetness, it does not create cavities. The content, lactic acid in the yogurt helps to protect gums and keep your teeth healthy. The antibiotic content promotes tooth health and safeguards against eroding tooth enamel, the main cause of decay. Individuals, who eat at least half a cup of yogurt daily, have a lower risk of getting the severe periodontal disease than those who do not consume it.

Good Bacteria: Yogurt is an excellent food and works great for our bodies. If you take antibiotic medicine for any sickness; it washes away the good bacteria completely from our intestines. Ayurvedic practitioners advise us to consume half a cup of yogurt every day for two weeks to compensate it .

Helps Sleeplessness: If one eats yogurt with a big pinch of black pepper and a teaspoon of fennel seed powder for two weeks, one will feel relaxed mentally and physically which promotes sleeping well at night.

Raw Milk Yogurt: Some people think they are doing an excellent job by feeding their bodies' raw milk yogurt and believe that has more value. Please pay attention; learn to bring beneficial bacteria into your body. When we make yogurt, we heat up to a boiling point, reduce it to a lukewarm level and add a tablespoon of yogurt and keep covered the whole night. Next morning it is ready, and we refrigerate it. Raw milk possesses E. coli and salmonella which cause problems to the body. To prevent sickness, we have to boil the milk to kill the harmful pathogens. Remember, boiling or pasteurization of milk does not destroy beneficial probiotics.

NOTE: - Though yogurt is one of the best foods on this earth, some people, who suffer from asthma, pneumonia, cough, breathing problems, any blood condition, and fever, should not consume it. If you eat it under these circumstances, it can increase the problem, and you may suffer more. So please stay away from yogurt. We have yogurt for breakfast or lunch but do not eat it at night, because as per my Nature Cure doctors, "It is not favorable to our health."

Zucchini

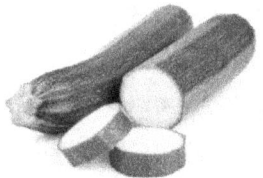

Zucchini is the world's healthiest vegetable. Being a little creative, you can cook it in many ways and create various delicious and savory dishes. It is full of nutrients, vitamins and minerals which are essential for our health. It is a light food, so we can consume a full bowl whether it is cooked, roasted, sautéed, steamed or grilled. Its essential contents of fiber and pectin help us lose weight, too.

Diabetes: Zucchini has an abundance of Vitamin B complex which is beneficial to diabetic patients. When the human body cannot metabolize and regulate blood sugar level, diabetes sneaks in. If you consume this vegetable on a daily basis, it safeguards from this condition. Even if you are a patient of diabetes type-2, eating zucchini will stabilize your blood sugar. You will lose weight because of its fiber, and it will help regulate your metabolism.

Eye Health: Zucchini is a significant source of Vitamin A, which is beneficial for eye health. It promotes the development of cells in your eyes. It also aids in removing the puffy bags around the eyes, and improves vision. Its beta carotene with Vitamin C and other important compounds such as antioxidants assist in protecting our eyes.

Lowers Blood Pressure: Potassium and magnesium which are present in zucchini, contribute to lowering blood pressure levels in the body. Regular consumption of this plant promotes to reduce high blood pressure and hypertension. If your blood pressure is stable, there are fewer chances of having a stroke or a heart attack.

Lose Weight: My cousin was here for a month, and I kept bugging him to lose some weight as he got big. A week before he was to leave for India, his blood pressure increased. I got his medicine to lower it and requested him that he eat lots of green vegetables in his daily meals. He went back and after six months he sent me an email saying, "Thanks for the tips you gave to me in the US. All this time, I have been eating green vegetables like zucchini, squash, and cabbage and I have lost 13 lbs." As zucchini contains water and it is a light food, it helps one to lose weight. Be little creative and prepare this vegetable the way you like and eat it every day. tends to push out more fluid (urine and toxins),

Lowers Cholesterol: It includes dietary fiber that contributes to the lowering of the cholesterol level in our digestive system. It also assists in preventing cholesterol buildup or oxidizing in the blood vessels because of its high levels of Vitamin A and Vitamin C; thus safeguarding us against infections.

Heart Health: Zucchini includes folic acid, which is a vital vitamin that helps to break down the harmful amino acids and guarantees against blood clotting. This plant also contains magnesium which helps reduce the risk of stroke and heart attack. The antioxidant compound in it also promotes lowering cholesterol and high blood pressure; thus aiding heart health.

It Is Anti-ageing: Free radicals cause fine lines to appear on the face and the body's skin. They cause age spots and wrinkles on the face. Regular consumption of zucchini can help slow down the signs of aging to some extent. This plant is an excellent source of crucial vitamins which are called the powerhouse of antioxidants and assist us in maintaining a healthy skin and a healthy body. It also includes manganese which produces Choline, the amino acid which aids in collagen formation; thus healing our wounds and keeping our skin healthy and toned.

Prevents Cancer: It possesses a high level of fiber that contributes to preventing harmful toxins from accumulating in the colon and makes soft bowel movements. Vitamin C and Vitamin A are vital anti-oxidizing agents that aids in destroying the dangerous bacteria which can lead to different kinds of cancers, especially prostate Cancer. To prevent cancer problems we all should consume this vegetable lavishly.

Gout and Arthritis: Gout and arthritis are painful conditions due to the inflammation of the joints. Eating zucchini aids in frequent urination, thus pushing out excessive uric acid from the body. Its anti-inflammatory and carotenoids can safeguard against the effects of inflammation and uric acid. It is also high in Omega-3 fatty acids which ease the pain of your knees and other joints. Ayurvedic practitioners advise us to plan a proper vegetarian diet which includes an increased consumption of green vegetables and fruits. Zucchini comes under the category of alkaline foods that act against the uric acid in our joints; thus relieving its symptoms. Its powerful properties of antioxidant Vitamins, C, Vitamin A and with copper help prevent the development of many inflammatory disorders like asthma, rheumatoid arthritis, gout, and osteoarthritis.

Hydrates The Skin: As we all know, Zucchini has a high water content which hydrates our skin. Water is so beneficial for our skin, it cleanses our digestive system, exfoliates the skin, and flushes out toxins from our bodies. Its regular consumption promotes the restoration the moisture of our skin, giving us a fair and glowing skin. I have heard rubbing its inner portion on puffy bags around the eyes helps ease the swollen part, but I have never tried it.

Hair Growth: Zucchini is rich in Vitamin A, and Vitamin C. Vitamin A assists in protecting hair from free radicals. If you do not consume this valuable nutrient, in your body, the hair becomes dry and starts falling out. Vitamin C is equally important in maintaining healthy collagen and in nourishing the follicles. Just incorporate it into your diet any way you want to.

Acknowledgements

"Thanks a lot to my husband Shiv Abrol and my lovely daughters Shivani, Seema, and Simi for helping me and being there for me all the time. Thanks to my dear friend Cynthia for her heavenly help."

Tiny precautions and simple meals help keep your body free of disease.

Life is not fun, but still beautiful.

Sit in solitude to find abundance.

Have patience, time is a great healer.

Community service is the service to the Lord.

Forgive others, let go and liberate yourself.

Have a firm faith in the NAME you believe in.

Indulging in gossip depletes your vital energy.

To enjoy the present, make peace with your past.

Happiness is instilled within, stop looking outside.

Never forget you are HIS creation, you are precious.

Before you sleep, thank Him for the blessed gift of life.

What people think about you is none of your business.

Make three people smile each day to enjoy the present.

Life is too short to nurture jealousy, hatred and revenge.

Find a purpose of your life and seek the guidance of the Lord.

Do not try to win every argument. Agreeing to disagree is calming.

Life is your personal journey and it is all about you. Do not involve others.

Consume one ounce of nuts daily to increase your vitality and longevity.

Drink 40 oz. of water daily first thing in the morning to detoxify your body.

Consumption of plant based food is much better than manufactured food.

All the berries, leafy greens, vegetables, and fruits help you to stay skinny.

"Eat a healthy meal always that cultivates your body, nurtures your mind, and nourishes your Soul."

-Sudesh-